AIDS:

The "Perfect" Disease

By

Jerry Leonard

ISBN: 0-7596-6808-6 (e-book)
ISBN: 0-7596-6809-4 (Paperback)

This book is printed on acid free paper.

1st Books - rev. 07/10/02

AIDS: The "Perfect" Disease

The Common Thread of Government Experimentation in the Acquired Immunodeficiency and Gulf War Syndromes

Jerry Leonard

If I were a devil creating a malicious virus to cause the most problems for the human race, the virus would be AIDS. The virus has found the Achilles' heel of the immune system.[1]

—Luc Montagnier

Thus the AIDS epidemic is providing a natural experiment on a massive scale from which much can be learned about the role of immunosuppression in the development of cancer.[2]

Some of the countries most affected by AIDS epidemics are projected to have zero or near-zero population growth, because of the higher mortality rates combined with low projected fertility rates.[3]

It is not inconceivable that we will, one of these days, have a visitation from a "super flu," perhaps much more virulent than the famous killer of 1918-1920. ... But what if a much more lethal strain should start going in the starving, more crowded population a few years from now? This could happen naturally or through the escape of a special strain created for biological warfare.[4]

—*Paul Ehrlich, 1968*

Over the next 10 years in Africa, AIDS is expected to kill more people and orphan more children than all the wars of the 20th century combined.[5]

—*Bill Clinton, 1999*

Preface

The AIDS epidemic is a larger, more sophisticated version of documented experiments conducted on human subjects.

An outrageous statement? Without question. One that contradicts or has not appeared in the popular press? Of course. But is it true? You be the judge. This study will suggest there is more to the AIDS epidemic than we are being told. Moreover, a case can be made that it was intentionally introduced into human populations for cancer research and national security purposes, and it is not far-fetched to suggest that AIDS is proving highly beneficial to both of those communities.

Consider these theories:

- AIDS was made possible by the cancer research establishment's documented creation and testing of immunosuppressive viruses similar to HIV as a tool in the development of human cancer vaccines.
- AIDS and the tragic epidemic of human cancer it has caused are the legacy of increasingly sophisticated and expansive experiments *that were designed to deliberately induce cancer in humans using monkey tumor and cancer-causing viruses.*[6]
- The cancer research establishment, which was intertwined with and funded by the national security establishment, was used as a tool to implement an international biowarfare effort using HIV in the Third World. [7]

These theories are not as far-fetched as you would believe. HIV is providing fantastic benefits to both the cancer research[8] and the national security establishments. And it is an ideal vehicle for the elimination of human cancer through the development of vaccines and for cutting out the "human cancer"[9] of population growth through biowarfare.

This study will tell you why.

Introduction

...scientists saw in the tragedy of the AIDS epidemic an extraordinary opportunity to study the interplay of viruses, an impaired immune system and the development of cancer. In a way, AIDS research was an extension of the war on cancer that the Government declared in 1971.[10]

The AIDS epidemic, caused by a mysterious monkey immunosuppressive virus that suddenly crossed into humans and caused an epidemic of cancer,[11] did not catch the entire medical community off guard. Quite the contrary. For decades prior to the AIDS outbreak, cancer virus researchers had been creating, manipulating, studying and testing immunosuppressive viruses[12] with selective immune system damaging and cancer-causing properties remarkably similar to AIDS.[13] *Moreover, several of these immunosuppressive viruses (including those from monkeys and humans) were being grown in human cell cultures shortly before the AIDS epidemic broke out in humans.*

These unique viruses were created as part of the U.S. government's war on cancer in a crash program to develop vaccines. These experimental immunosuppressive viruses, which were isolated from mice, cats, cows and monkeys in the 1960s and 1970s, were successfully used to destructively manipulate the immune systems of a variety of lab animals as a means of controllably *increasing* susceptibility to cancer.[14] *This research was conducted so that scientists could learn more about precisely how immune system dysfunction contributed to cancer growth.* The innovative research with these novel immunosuppressive viruses provided valuable information on the role that various components of the immune system played in cancer prevention and aided the development of various means of manipulating the immune system to prevent cancer in animals.

Interestingly, the selective immune system damage caused by the AIDS epidemic in humans is supplying cancer researchers with invaluable data eerily similar to that which they obtained in the 1970s by deliberately injecting the immunosuppressive viruses they created in animal test subjects. This is so because the cancer epidemic initiated by AIDS[15] is providing observant researchers a wealth of invaluable data about how cancer grows—from its earliest to its latest phases—in human subjects with selectively impaired immune systems.[16] By constructing huge databases on how cancer grows in AIDS patients as their immune systems systematically degrade, researchers are quietly finding such powerful clues as to the mechanisms behind the increased susceptibility to cancer in human AIDS patients—especially those cancers thought to be caused by viruses—that many are now confidently predicting the imminent development of human cancer vaccines. Such a phenomenal development would mirror similar progress made earlier in animal cancer research with immunosuppressive and cancer viruses.[17]

It is at this point that a terrible question must be asked: Could HIV, and the epidemic of human cancers and death resulting from it, be the result of a sinister cross-species experiment with a monkey cancer virus designed as a means of intentionally inducing cancer in human subjects as a research and diagnostic tool in the development of human cancer vaccines? If so, was such an experiment modeled after decades of similar animal experiments in which well-characterized immunosuppressive viruses similar to HIV were injected in test subjects so that cancer researchers could monitor the progress of induced cancer growth as the animals' immune systems deteriorated? And was this why researchers were growing monkey and human immunosuppressive viruses in human cell cultures, determining the pathogenic effects on T-cells, shortly before HIV began to destroy T-cells in the immune systems of human populations?[18]

Unfortunately, there are numerous disturbing precedents indicating that cancer researchers would do this very thing. These precedents supply deeply disquieting evidence consistent with the terrifying hypothesis that the AIDS epidemic, caused by a simian virus that has resulted in an unprecedented international human cancer epidemic, is the result of the wider application of shockingly unethical and dangerous human cancer experiments with simian cancer viruses conducted throughout the 1950s and 60s.

As will be discussed in greater detail in a later section, in one set of these cross-species cancer vaccine experiments, immunosuppressed rats *and humans* were given the same set of cancer-inducing virus injections so that the tumors that developed in each species could be systematically compared.[19] In a similar set of such immunosuppressive experiments, *tumors were deliberately induced in human subjects as a result of injections with monkey tumor and cancer viruses, so that researchers could compare the resultant human tumors with those that grew in the monkeys.*[20] As an extension of this type of work, in the 1970s, shortly before AIDS began in human populations, researchers began combining primate cancer viruses that had been injected in human subjects *with primate immunodeficiency viruses* in human cell cultures.[21]

For example, while the public is completely ignorant of this fact, *simian immunosuppressive viruses* (SIVs) such as the Mason Pfizer Monkey Virus—one of 3 types of SIV[22]—were available to researchers as early as 1970, when the virus was grown in cell cultures.[23] Well before AIDS, the Mason Pfizer Monkey Virus (MPMV) was shown to induce immunodeficiency states in monkeys in the early 1970s,[24,25] as well as the 1980s.[26] Even more provocative is the fact that cancer researchers were coaxing this immunosuppressive monkey virus to grow in human cells in the late 1970s—just before HIV broke out in human populations and caused an epidemic of sarcoma. In these experiments, MPMV was mixed with SV40—a monkey cancer virus (which had already been injected in humans to cause cancer) and the Rous sarcoma virus in *human* cell cultures.[27] Since HIV is thought to be caused by an SIV, it is amazing that these intriguing pre-AIDS experiments have not been publicized.

The national security establishment, which worked closely with the viral cancer research community, is likewise not a disinterested party in the AIDS epidemic. While cancer researchers are benefiting from the selective depopulation of certain cells in the immune systems of HIV victims, it could be argued that *the national security planners in fact are benefiting from the resultant selective destruction of human populations.* This depopulation effect is fulfilling national security goals for the Third World, where 90% of AIDS deaths occur and where 95% of world population growth occurs, that were outlined in classified national security planning documents shortly before AIDS broke out.

The latter section of this study will examine the hypothesized linkage between cancer research and the interests of the national security community. *Specifically, evidence will be presented to support the thesis that the AIDS epidemic was deliberately started as an exercise in biowarfare conducted under the cover of a human cancer experiment.* This would explain why the HIV epidemic is selectively depopulating regions of the globe that the national security establishment had targeted for depopulation in the 1970s as a means of maintaining access to resources in the developing world. Additionally, the "cancer vaccine experiment" theory of the origin of AIDS could also explain not only why the AIDS virus selectively depopulates the exact components of the immune system that cancer researchers had been targeting for decades prior to AIDS but why homosexual populations are disproportionately infected by HIV and rare cancers. And finally, there is credible evidence that AIDS vaccine research vehicles have a linkage to the Gulf War Syndrome.

Uncle Sam's Guinea Pigs

On the other hand, the effectiveness of the substances on individuals at all social levels, high and low, native American and foreign, is of great significance and testing has been performed on a variety of individuals within these categories.[28]

Alert students of current events over the last several decades have read, through various outlets of the mainstream media and numerous congressional and presidential committees, a continuous stream of evidence implicating the U.S. government in an uninterrupted program of massive, covert experimentation on its citizens. This protracted program of dangerous experimentation is breathtaking both in its scale and its complete lack of accountability.

Recent headlines have revealed that throughout the 1950s and '60s, thousands of citizens were quietly and systematically exposed to dangerous levels of radiation for experimental purposes. A presidential commission appointed by the Clinton administration published a massive 900-page exposé of an extensive, decades-long set of radiation experiments covertly conducted on an unwitting citizenry.[29] Many of these radiation experiments were conducted under the pretext of cancer research in order to develop or evaluate national security-related weapons systems.

The 4,000 known experiments[30] conducted under the umbrella of these unethical tests included the following: administering radioactive pills to pregnant women;[31] giving children cereal that was intentionally

1

contaminated with radioactive iron and calcium;[32] exposing soldiers to radiation at ground-zero after atomic blasts;[33] and exposing populated civilian areas to radiation, both through deliberate releases of atomic clouds from rockets[34] and intentional leaks at atomic facilities.[35]

* * *

Documents declassified in the 1970s revealed that, in parallel with these radiation experiments, the government had been systematically experimenting on its citizens and especially its soldiers (again, for decades, starting in the 1940s) with dangerous drugs and chemicals. These included deadly nerve gases, candidate mind control drugs such as LSD and incapacitating agents.[36] Like the covert radiation experiments, some of these chemical warfare tests were conducted under the pretext of cancer research. (Several of these tests were conducted on U.S. soldiers in "gas chamber" experiments at American military bases under the guidance of Nazi chemical warfare specialists recruited after the Second World War.[37])

This experimentation on soldiers may have more bearing on current events than is apparent at first glance. Questions have been raised in the popular press,[38] medical literature and a Senate investigation on the link between the Gulf War Syndrome now afflicting many U.S. soldiers and such dangerous, ongoing government experimentation.

In fact, the most recent example of this experimentation was the vaccines and unproved chemical warfare countermeasures (drugs) dispensed to hundreds of thousands of unwitting[39] troops involved in the Gulf War mobilization.[40]

This government-sanctioned experimentation[41] has justifiably outraged members of Congress[42] as well as veterans. Additionally, and disturbingly, this experimentation has also been linked to one of several identified Gulf War syndromes in a medical study conducted by researchers from the University of Texas Southwestern Medical Center.[43] This study, published in the *Journal of the American Medical Association*, found that some of the debilitating syndromes experienced by Gulf War veterans may be due to an artificially increased sensitivity to chemicals used in the Gulf War as a result of the administration of an experimental drug known as pyridostigmine bromide. This study bolstered the findings of the Rockefeller Committee back in 1994.[44] The dangers of an increased sensitivity to normally harmless chemicals such as pesticides or dangerous chemicals such as nerve gases, as a result of the administration of this experimental drug were warned of in the committee's report on Gulf War Syndrome.[45]

Proper safeguards were blatantly disregarded in the administration of the drug. Individuals who were known to be dangerously hypersensitive to it were not screened out before its indiscriminate administration.[46] Additionally, the government gave these experimental drugs to female soldiers despite the fact that no tests had been conducted to determine the effects on healthy women or women who were on medication such as birth control pills.[47] Given these facts, it is not surprising that an estimated 50% of those who took the experimental drugs experienced side effects. For some of these, the side effects have apparently been catastrophic.

An added irony is that the experimental drugs were not even effective against the type of nerve gas that U.S. intelligence claimed that the Iraqis were about to use. They were designed to be used against the gases soman or tabun, not against sarin, which American intelligence deemed likely to be used.[48] *In fact, PB makes humans more susceptible to sarin than they would be without the treatment.*[49]

After years of cover-up, it came to light that possibly 100,000 U.S. troops were exposed to sarin *as a result of the Defense Department's March 1991 destruction of an Iraqi chemical weapons depot containing nerve gases.*[50,51]

Other Texas researchers have found disturbing evidence of governmental biological warfare experimentation on this same group of Gulf War soldiers. In this case, the researchers were Drs. Garth and Nancy Nicolson, formerly the Chair in Cancer Research at the University of Texas M.D. Anderson Cancer Center in Houston and an instructor in biophysics at Baylor College of Medicine, respectively.[52] These researchers found what they believe to be a biological warfare agent known as *mycoplasma fermentans* in the cells of many Gulf War vets they've examined. As a result of their own daughter, herself a Gulf War vet, coming down with symptoms typical of those with the Gulf War Syndrome, the Nicolsons devised a method of treating this particular syndrome with antibiotics. (Curiously, this cure was based on Nancy's experience treating her own disease, which had caused similar symptoms years earlier.) This successful treatment caught the attention of the Veterans Affairs Department, which began a multi-city investigation into the effectiveness of the Nicolsons' treatment for Gulf War Syndrome.

Interestingly enough, the Nicolsons have reported finding a genetically engineered version of the mycoplasma in U.S. soldiers, which allegedly includes a gene from HIV, called GP-120.[53] While the Nicolsons believe this organism may have been engineered to allow it to destructively target certain immune cells, others have speculated that this infectious organism was designed and unleashed on soldiers as part of an investigation into an HIV vaccine, some versions of which use this same gene.[54]

Evidence that the immunological abnormalities associated with the Gulf War Syndrome are related to government experimentation with AIDS vaccines continues to mount. *Insight Magazine* has published a shocking exposé, which confirms that powerful and dangerous synthetic chemicals created for use in highly experimental vaccines, including AIDS vaccines, have been found in sick Gulf War vets with the Gulf War Syndrome.[55] (Notably, troops who received the experimental vaccines, but never went overseas during the war, have become sick with the Gulf War Syndrome. This eliminates any chemical or biological warfare use by the Iraqis as a culprit in these cases.) Using a new process developed at Tulane Medical School, researchers have identified a synthetic vaccine additive called squalene in the blood of many sick Gulf War vets. The synthetic form of this potent chemical, which has been officially approved only in very limited human experiments, is not naturally occurring.

It is only known to be manufactured at a *military* hospital—Walter Reed. After years of denials, the Pentagon has reluctantly admitted that this chemical and this hospital have been involved in a previously unknown AIDS vaccine experiment in Thailand.[56] However, the government has denied the chemical was used on Gulf War troops.

Did U.S. government experimentation with a highly potent immune system altering pharmaceutical product result in the strange immune system abnormalities associated with Gulf War Syndrome?[57] Such a scenario might explain the strange manner in which sick soldiers were treated by the government after the war. As related by *Insight*:

> Scores of them [Gulf War vets] were placed in Walter Reed's special HIV ward and isolated even from their doctors by personnel brought in from special DOD units to conduct medical evaluations based on AIDS-related symptoms. Many of these patients not only never learned what the specialist teams discovered, or for that matter what they failed to find, but they were required to submit to further semiannual HIV-examination testing procedures for many years without explanation.

(It was the sending out of Gulf War vets' blood samples for testing related to this monitoring program at Walter Reed that led to *Insight's* exposé, as researchers at Tulane Medical School, using a proprietary process they developed, found the experimental chemical in some of the samples they retained.)

Rather than simply investigate the scenario that experimental vaccines with squalene have contributed to the Gulf War Syndrome, the government is apparently in full cover-up mode. It has not only classified information related to the experimental vaccines given the troops, but has also classified information regarding the use of the experimental agent squalene used in the experimental HIV vaccines overseas.

In a like manner, the British government is also refusing to divulge what was in the vaccine given to its troops. Like their American counterparts, British troops who did not serve in the Gulf, but who did receive the vaccines, are testing positive for the vaccine additive. As the Paul Brown writing in the British *Guardian* recently summarized:

> The illness known as Gulf war syndrome looks likely to have been caused by an illegal vaccine "booster" given by the Ministry of Defence to protect soldiers against biological weapons, according to the results of a new series of tests.

Continuing, Brown noted:

> The evidence could be devastating for the Ministry of Defence which is being sued for damages by 1,900 British veterans. If they show they were injected with an illegal substance, the damages could be astronomical. The ministry has refused to reveal what was in the injections.[58]

* * *

Jerry Leonard

Neither of these two theories for the source of the Gulf War Syndrome—experimental chemical treatments with pyrodostigmine bromide and experimental HIV vaccines—should be dismissed out of hand. The large-scale, covert governmental testing of chemical/biological warfare agents and treatments on soldiers would hardly be unprecedented. Scientists at Fort Detrick in Maryland, for example, began a decades-long program of systematically exposing military personnel to various pathogens almost immediately following World War II.[59]

In addition to Gulf War Syndrome, there are alarming links between the Acquired Immunodeficiency Syndrome (AIDS) and ongoing government experimentation revolving around vaccine programs. Although there are similarities in the purposes behind and the methods by which the Gulf War and Acquired Immunodeficiency Syndromes are suspected to have been initiated (vaccines), there are differences in the end result. In the case of the Gulf War Syndrome, an agent allegedly added to the vaccines designed to *heighten* the immune system response as an HIV vaccine research tool has been implicated in various pathologies. In the case of the AIDS epidemic, it is proposed that a contaminating agent in the vaccines was designed to selectively *destroy* components of the immune system as a cancer vaccine research tool. (This type of experimentation is referred to as immunosuppressive research.)

Immunosuppression as a Tool in Cancer Virus Research

A major goal in immunology has been to find a means of selectively abolishing an individual's potential to mount an immune response to certain antigens, while preserving responsiveness to others.[60]

It is a little-known fact that *selective immune system damage* (or immunosuppression), such as that caused by HIV, while often devastating to its victims, is a medically useful phenomenon that has historically been both exploited *and created* by medical researchers for experimental purposes. For example, in addition to its well-known use in organ transplantation research, exotic forms of immunosuppression have been both developed and used by medical researchers for decades in a bizarre and dangerous line of government-financed experimentation known as "cancer transplantation" research. Experiments conducted and published during this research included the successful transplantation of cancer from man-to-man, man-to-monkey and monkey-to-man.

This research was conducted as a component of an ambitious, long-running research effort designed to develop human cancer vaccines. It involved transplanting cancer cells or cancer viruses from one organism to another to observe how the immune system reacted to prevent cancer growth in the recipient organism. It was hoped that, by watching how experimental cancer *transplants* were or were not rejected in various test subjects, researchers could gain

9

knowledge of how humans rejected *natural* forms of cancer. It was further hoped that this knowledge would be directly applicable to the development of human cancer vaccines.

In numerous experiments of this type, which were designed to provide insight into the precise mechanisms of subsequent cancer rejection or growth, cancer transplants were injected into organisms of varying immune system health. *It was in order to generate organisms with various immune system defects for these studies that numerous means of inducing immune system deficiencies (or immunodeficiencies) were eventually developed.*

One type of immunosuppression—caused by immunosuppressive *viruses* with properties similar to HIV[61]—has been used by cancer researchers for approximately thirty years now[62] as a novel immunological tool to intentionally increase the susceptibility of animals to cancer virus injections.[63] (These viruses were invented to test the hypothesis that immunosuppression aided cancer growth. Or, as it was stated in one technical paper, "that transient immune impairment may serve as an important contributing factor in tumor proliferation."[64]) It is this line of research involving the sophisticated use of immunosuppressive viruses for cancer experiments that has many curious trails leading to the human epidemic of AIDS.

The Goals and Methods of the Viral Cancer Research Establishment

In order to fully understand why immunosuppressive viruses capable of inducing diseases such as AIDS in mice[65] were developed long ago by the cancer research establishment, one must gain an understanding of the overarching goals of the cancer virus research community *and* the specific methods developed to achieve these goals. These goals included the following:

1) Proving that "cancer viruses" were capable of inducing human cancers
2) Proving that a faulty immune system was instrumental in determining susceptibility to these cancer viruses, and
3) Demonstrating that vaccines could be created to assist the immune system in the fight against these alleged human cancer viruses—resulting in a long-sought cure for cancer.[66]

As mentioned above, one of the chief methods that has been used in attempts to prove these "cancer virus" theories includes the controlled exposure of test subjects to cancer agents in combination with artful manipulation of the immune system. By systematically exposing animal and human subjects of varying immune system health to potential cancer viruses,[67] researchers hoped to determine not only whether such viruses could cause cancer but also what factors determined susceptibility to these cancer-causing viruses. By gaining a thorough understanding of the causes of cancer, researchers hoped to be able to completely control cancer growth—creating it or stopping it on command.[68]

To this end, numerous experiments were carried out in which experimental subjects were exposed to cancer agents in conjunction with treatments that were designed either to *detract from* or *enhance* their existing immune system capabilities. Such work involving the suppression or stimulation of the immune system promised to identify any immune system defects that rendered animals and humans more susceptible to cancer viruses *and* to identify methods of compensating for such defects that might ultimately render humans immune to cancer viruses.

Enhancing the Immune System Response to Cancer

These experiments involve the use of *cancer injections* in human subjects in attempts designed to understand and fight cancer. Such experiments—aimed at using cancer injections to *enhance* the human immune system's ability to reject cancer—have a long and sordid history. In one early and primitive experiment of this type (from the 1920s), a human patient with cancer was injected with human leukemia cells from another patient in an attempt to stimulate her immune system to fight cancer.[69] In later experiments of this type, a researcher injected cancer patients with their own cancer cells, as well as those from other cancer patients, in attempts to inoculate them against their own cancer.[70]

Increasingly sophisticated experiments of this type—designed to enhance the human immune response to controlled amounts of cancer agents—

continued for decades. In one series of such experiments, published by a tireless and unscrupulous researcher named Chester Southam, patients were given transplants of two different types of cells. Specifically, patients were given injections of *cancer cells* in combination with injections of *immune system cells* (such as leukocytes from healthy donors), which were designed to assist their immune systems in rejecting the cancer cells. In these "immunotherapy" tests using potentially deadly cancer cell injections, researchers compared the ability of these leukocyte transplants to assist the patients in rejecting cancer transplants, relative to patients who didn't receive the leukocyte transplants (but who did receive cancer cell transplants).[71]

Other tests of this nature were conducted in which human subjects were given injections of cancer cells in conjunction with various treatments designed to increase their ability to reject cancer. In one case, again involving Southam, humans were injected with live cancer cells in combination with injections of live viruses. It was hoped that the live viruses would stimulate the subjects' immune systems and thereby enhance their ability to reject the cancer cells.[72] The goal was to measure and compare tumor formation in the human cancer cell transplant recipients between the patients who received the viral co-injections and those who didn't receive them.

During these experiments, Southam regretted the fact the viruses he was injecting with the cancer were too readily rejected by his human subjects. For example, in one of his earliest published experiments involving the injection of promising anti-cancer viruses in humans, Southam found that his subjects' immune systems quickly acquired the ability to reject repeat injections of the "anti-tumor" viruses he was using. Southam voiced the hope that, to overcome this problem, "methods might be developed by which antiviral immunity could be destroyed, thus permitting re-infection with the same virus."[73] Southam's wish that immunosuppressive techniques would be successfully developed and employed in cancer research was eventually fulfilled and such techniques were used extensively in animal model experiments.[74]

Immunocompetence through Immunocompromise

Experiments designed to help human subjects reject cancer, while sometimes apparently successful, were not very reliable or repeatable. Consequently, researchers set out to determine exactly what agents were responsible for human cancer (for example, viruses) and exactly which immune system components might be gainfully manipulated to prevent or cure cancer due to these agents. One component of this research involved "immunosuppressive" cancer research in animals.

Immunosuppressive research was a supplement to the attempts at "jump-starting" a patient's immune system response to cancer. In this research, in contrast to procedures designed to aid the immune system's response to cancer, scientists developed methods to intentionally and selectively *inhibit* an experimental subject's ability to mount an immune response to cancer.

By selectively eliminating certain classes of immune system cells (such as leukocytes) and watching how diseases such as cancer developed in their absence, researchers hoped to gain insight as to how these cells helped prevent disease in healthy subjects. The idea was that if cancer susceptibility could be made to artificially *increase* when a certain immune system component was purposely disabled or "knocked out" through these "immunodepressive" techniques, then it might be assumed that this component played a major role in cancer prevention. (In other words, researchers attempted to identify the various immune system components required for health by selectively destroying them and watching for pathology.)

Once the immune system components required for cancer prevention were identified through this destructive process, more focused and effective techniques might be devised in follow-up experiments to *bolster* these specific components as an "immunologic" means of cancer prevention.[75] This approach effectively represented a two-step process to cancer prevention, consisting of 1) the identification of immune system defects that aided cancer growth, followed by 2) the compensation for these defects in those who were afflicted with them.

The use of controlled forms of immune system damage, or immunosuppression, as a means of deliberately and precisely impairing the immune system to increase susceptibility to cancer viruses proved a successful strategy for "dissecting" the immune response to cancer in animals. Early forms of selective immunosuppression, which were capable of eliminating classes of immune system cells (such as T-cells) in mice while leaving others (such as B-cells) intact, included the use of surgical procedures such as the removal the thymus (a procedure known as a "thymectomy"). Numerous combinations of chemical agents and radiation treatments were also used to induce immunosuppressive states in lab animals as a means of controllably increasing cancer growth due to cancer virus injections.[76] Eventually, viruses and then methods developed in genetic engineering research were used to create laboratory animals with precisely impaired immune systems (so-called "knockouts") so that the effectiveness of the immune response to various "challenging agents" could be measured in these deliberately impaired animals and compared with healthy counterparts.[77]

Thus, by measuring the immune response of healthy and immunosuppressed test animals to cancer injections, researchers could evaluate the role of various immune system components in preventing cancer. Once immune system defects that led to cancer growth were identified, researchers could then evaluate the effectiveness of vaccines designed to assist these components in rejecting cancer. For example, after years of experiments determined that the CD4 T-cells were critical for fighting cancer in animals, researchers are now spending enormous amounts of time "priming" these cells to fight various forms of cancer. This successful line of research[78] is still being actively pursued.

In one set of these T-cell studies, researchers found that the growth of cancer transplants could be reduced through the use of a cancer "vaccine" consisting of killed *Corynebacterium parvum* in combination with immunosuppressive treatments.[79] The immunosuppressive techniques used for this set of experiments consisted of surgically removing the thymus in young mice, in combination with radiation and chemical treatments designed to deliberately reduce the T-cell response to cancer transplants. The degree to which the T-cell response had been deliberately suppressed was measured by observing the response of the test animals to calibrated antigens (the typical response to these antigens was well known from previous experiments in healthy mice). As a result of the immunosuppressive treatments and subsequent exposure to well-known antigens, researchers verified that the animals "had been made severely deficient in respect of their T-cell population." Cancer growth due to the transplants could then be correlated with the immune system stimulation due to the experimental vaccine and the degree to which the T-cell response had been impaired.[80]

As a result of these experimental methods, which could be used to effect a reduction in cancer susceptibility as well as dissect the immune system, researchers had a novel tool for determining exactly which components of the immune system were stimulated by the vaccine and why cancer was surprisingly decreased in the immunosuppressed animals.[81] The role of the T-cell response in preventing certain forms of cancer could thus be evaluated.

Myriad experiments of this type have been conducted in which mice were injected with cancer viruses and cells after being immunosuppressed through chemical, surgical, viral and genetic engineering techniques.

While primitive immunosuppressive techniques using surgery, radiation and chemicals could provide some clues as to the exact nature of the immune response to cancer, greater refinement in the ability to target subclasses of immune system cells was needed. Such precision was required to determine exactly which immune system cells were preventing cancer— either directly or indirectly (through interactions with other immune system cells).

As cited earlier, viral immunosuppression using RNA leukemia viruses developed in mice[82] and cats[83] was an additional method of inducing such selective immunosuppression, which was used successfully by the cancer research community as far back as the 1960s.[84] This method of employing viruses to induce immunosuppression provided a "viral scalpel" with which certain immune system products (such as T-cells) could be selectively eliminated as a means of deliberately increasing the susceptibility of lab animals to co-injections of cancer viruses.

In these experiments, researchers would inject mice with both sarcoma viruses and immunosuppressive leukemia viruses.[85] Once the leukemia viruses damaged the immune systems of the experimental mice, researchers measured the resulting cancer susceptibility (due to the sarcoma viruses) in the leukemia virus-impaired test subjects.[86]

The differences in cancer susceptibility between the intentionally immunosuppressed mice and the healthy mice used in these experiments provided a "window" on the immune system reaction to cancer and helped researchers identify the critical immune system components involved in preventing cancer.[87]

After these critical components were identified using various types of immunosuppression in conjunction with cancer virus injections, researchers were able to work on preventive procedures for cancer by assisting the response of these identified components.[88]

This type of immunosuppressive research, in which scientists deliberately impaired the immune systems of animal test subjects with an array of immunosuppressive viruses,[89] aided researchers in their eventually successful attempts to create coveted vaccines to some cancer viruses in mice and cats.[90]

Human Experiments with Cancer Exploiting Immunosuppression

Experiments that exploited immune system impairment to increase susceptibility to cancer have also been conducted in humans. As shocking as this may sound, numerous well-documented studies have indeed been conducted and published over the past several decades in which human subjects with various forms of "natural" immunosuppression were systematically exposed to cancer-causing agents that induced tumors. In one set of experiments lasting over a decade, immune-impaired humans were given multiple injections of human cancer cells[91] to deliberately induce tumor formation.

Experiments of this type involving injections of cancer cells in human subjects were conducted on patients with varying immune system capabilities to measure how immune system health affected cancer growth. For example, hundreds of patients with advanced forms of cancer,[92] patients with advanced diseases other than cancer[93] and hundreds of healthy patients[94] (used as controls) were injected in these studies. The subjects' immune system reactions to cancer transplants were systematically measured in these experiments, as were the rates of formation and the sizes of the tumors, or "nodules," which formed as a result of the injections.

(These experiments with "transplantable cancers" had a two-fold purpose—to measure cancer susceptibility as a function of immune system health and to determine the feasibility of using controlled injections of cancer as potential human cancer vaccines. The researchers who conducted these experiments claimed success at both identifying immune system defects responsible for cancer growth[95] and at identifying an acquired immune response to cancer.[96])

These early cancer injection experiments, *which exploited naturally immunosuppressed human subjects* to monitor the human immune response to cancer cells, were followed up with similar experiments in which *researchers made use of "real time" destructive modification of human test subjects' immune systems.* In one set of experiments, a group of cancer patients undergoing immune system-altering chemotherapy was systematically given injections of six human cancer cell lines to see which types of cancer grew more effectively in the impaired human patients.[97] *In a parallel set of tests, immunosuppressed, or "conditioned," rats were given injections of the same cancer cells by the researchers so that the cancers which developed in the immunosuppressed human subjects could be directly compared with those that developed in the immunosuppressed animals.*

According to the authors of the paper describing this set of barbaric experiments (published in the medical journal *Cancer*), the tumors induced in the human patients were coldly reported to be "rather similar to the tumors produced in conditioned animals but had much less fibrous tissue."

AIDS: A Human Cancer Experiment?

Should the recent findings on mouse leukemia be applicable to the human disease, it would logically follow that in order to transmit experimentally human leukemia from man to man, newborn infants, and not adult individuals, would have to be inoculated, an obviously unthinkable experiment.[98]

The review of immunosuppressive cancer research raises some critical questions with respect to the explosive spread of the international epidemic of immunosuppression and cancer caused by the AIDS virus:

Could the human epidemic of HIV-induced immunosuppression and the associated epidemic of increased cancer susceptibility be the result of large-scale versions of these earlier human cancer transplant experiments—using the refinements perfected in animal studies with immunosuppressive viruses?

Could this be why the human epidemic of immunosuppression and cancer began only a few years after researchers began isolating and growing simian immunodeficiency viruses in human cells and mixing such viruses with animal cancer viruses and human cancer cells?

How Might An Alleged "AIDS Experiment" Be Conducted?

Scientists in the viral cancer research community developed various means of inducing immunosuppression in animals so that the role of the immune system in reacting to cancer injections could be more effectively studied. Much expertise was gained in causing precise forms of *selective* immunosuppression (for example, deliberately eliminating T-cell populations[99] or B-cell populations[100]) to increase susceptibility to cancer in animals.

Once breakthroughs were made in this immunosuppressive animal research, some researchers expressed the hope that these breakthroughs might be applied to human populations.[101]

Obviously, such experimentation with pathological viruses could not be *openly* conducted on a large scale in human populations. However, to *covertly* replicate the experiments routinely conducted on mice and cats, researchers could use existing vaccine programs as vehicles for human experimentation.[102] Vaccine programs supply the perfect vehicle for conducting such experiments—they provide a pretext for injecting humans with viruses as well as follow up studies to measure the effects of the injections. Legitimate vaccination campaigns could be used to quietly give a pre-selected group of human guinea pigs a *vaccine* secretly "contaminated" with immunosuppressive viruses.[103] Following this, researchers could then conduct long-term follow-up studies on the vaccine recipients to measure the progress of any cancer growth or the progress of other viral infections after immunosuppression "mysteriously" set in. By carefully monitoring how cancer grew in subjects whose immune systems progressively deteriorated,[104] invaluable clues might be obtained as to the mechanisms by which the human immune system prevented cancer.[105] These clues might provide enough information to allow preventive means against cancer (such as vaccines) to eventually be devised for humans—just as they were in animal cancer research.

AIDS in the U.S.:

Was such a calculated procedure followed in human populations? Could such malignant, pre-meditated planning and experimentation with immunosuppressive viruses explain the sudden and unprecedented outbreak of selective immunosuppression and cancer in homosexual populations *within the United States* in the early 1980s (shortly after AIDS-like diseases were created in monkeys)? Unfortunately there is much evidence consistent with this theory.

Consider this hypothesis: A core group of cancer researchers deliberately gave a pre-selected set of promiscuous homosexuals an experimental vaccine containing an immunosuppressive virus and, after immunosuppression set in, began to systematically monitor the cancers that developed in the vaccine recipients[106]—just as had been done in mouse and cat experiments in which test animals were monitored for cancer growth after they were given combinations of immunosuppressive leukemia and cancer viruses.

There is evidence to support this radical hypothesis. Promiscuous homosexuals *were* selectively targeted with an experimental vaccine against hepatitis B beginning in the late 1970s.[107] And the AIDS epidemic in promiscuous homosexuals began almost immediately after the first of these vaccine experiments.[108] It has been documented that recipients of this experimental hepatitis vaccine have been disproportionately afflicted with AIDS[109] *and* that immunosuppressed homosexuals are being targeted with numerous follow-up studies to monitor how cancer develops in immunosuppressed victims versus healthy populations.[110]

The suspect experimental hepatitis B vaccine given to homosexuals just prior to the AIDS epidemic appears to have been a subset of a proposed global cancer vaccine experiment administered by the World Health Organization.[111] It was thought that hepatitis B was the cause of a form of cancer called hepatocellular carcinoma and that by immunizing people against hepatitis, immunity to this form of cancer might be obtained.[112] Hepatitis B vaccination trials were conducted as a means of developing vaccines for use in these international hepatitis/cancer vaccine trials.[113]

Given the admitted experimental nature of this cancer vaccine effort and the useful immunosuppression subsequently associated with one branch of it, it seems logical to ask:

Was this direct attempt at cancer vaccination using the hepatitis B vaccine augmented through the addition of immunosuppressive viruses, as was done in experimental animal populations?[114] In other words, was there a hidden cancer vaccine experiment within the cancer vaccine experiment associated with the hepatitis B program?[115] Could this explain why immunosuppression in homosexual populations is proving so beneficial to cancer research?

The Source of the International AIDS Epidemic:

In addition to the AIDS outbreak in American homosexuals, there is evidence supporting the theory that the *international* HIV epidemic is also the result of a premeditated international "cancer vaccine" experiment implemented using existing vaccine programs associated with the World Health Organization (WHO).

While gay recipients of the hepatitis B/cancer vaccination program have been disproportionately stricken by the AIDS virus, according to a front page article in *The Times of London*, it is a segment of the recipients of the international smallpox vaccination administered by the WHO which have been disproportionately afflicted with AIDS in the developing world. As Pearce Wright summarized in the *Times*:

> The World Health Organization, which masterminded the 13 year campaign, is studying new scientific evidence suggesting that immunization with the smallpox vaccine Vaccinia awakened the unsuspected, dormant human immuno defence virus infection (HIV).[116]

The *Times* elaborated: "The smallpox vaccine theory would account for the position of each of the seven Central African states which top the league table of most affected countries; why Brazil became the most afflicted Latin American country; and how Haiti became the route for the spread of Aids to the U.S."

This development, in which human vaccine recipients in a WHO vaccination campaign have reportedly developed severe T-cell deficiencies as a result of a viral infection, is no less interesting in light of various statements that representatives of the WHO had made during the 1970s regarding the usefulness of vaccines and "immunological deficiency syndromes" in furthering human cancer research. For example, WHO representatives had made statements expressing their desire that the organization get involved in research with immunosuppressive viruses capable of selectively targeting T-cells.[117] (As noted above, these same researchers were optimistic that the immunosuppressive research conducted in animals could be usefully extended to human beings.[118]) Members of WHO had also recommended that experimental agents be placed in vaccines as a vehicle for measuring the human immune response on a global scale[119] (as a means of separating genetic from environmental determinants of immune system function). A report by a WHO study group had also recommended an international study of naturally immunosuppressed humans with *immunological deficiency syndromes* for cancer research purposes (this was prior to the emergence of the international Acquired Immunodeficiency Syndrome epidemic)![120]

Did WHO achieve all of these goals *simultaneously* by placing immunosuppressive agents in some of its vaccines, thereby creating a highly useful international epidemic of *acquired* immunodeficiency syndromes resulting from selective T-cell depletion?

The international immunosuppressive effects of the HIV virus are providing cancer researchers with a bonanza of invaluable data on the manner in which cancer grows in immunosuppressed human subjects (see below).[121] Such immunosuppression may ultimately provide answers as to whether many human cancers are the result of latent viruses that suddenly become pathogenic due to the destruction or impairment of the immune system.[122] This information will be vital to researchers working on the formulation of cancer vaccines.[123]

Precedents

Would the World Health Organization have conducted such a deadly experiment, on behalf of the cancer research establishment? A review of the documented history of government-sponsored immunosuppressive cancer research in human subjects may serve to remove natural doubts as to whether a "governmental" agency would have implemented such a premeditated experiment. Experiments similar to the one proposed in this article to explain the human AIDS epidemic have been conducted in human populations (albeit, on a smaller scale) by members of the government-funded cancer research establishment. In fact, *AIDS could be viewed—barring ethical considerations—as the culmination of decades of such documented research* designed to increase cancer susceptibility for research purposes by exploiting immunosuppression in humans and animals.

It is a fact that human "cancer vaccine" experiments involving deliberate infection with cancer have been routinely conducted for decades. Southam and his colleagues alone published dozens of papers in the 1950s and 1960s describing their systematic injection of "tumor transplants" in hundreds of unsuspecting healthy patients and patients who were immunosuppressed due to various illnesses and treatments.[124]

These published experiments on human subjects differ only slightly from the experiment proposed to explain the human AIDS epidemic and the associated cancer epidemic. The difference lies in the exploitation of *natural* forms of immunosuppression to increase cancer growth versus the deliberate *creation* of immunosuppression in human subjects for experimental purposes. Here, too, *published experiments indicate that cancer researchers have exploited real-time immune system destruction in conjunction with deliberate exposure of human subjects to cancer agents to deliberately increase and measure susceptibility to cancer.* Recall, for example, the experiments described in which cancer cell injections were used in human patients undergoing immunosuppressive chemotherapy.[125] Southam injected cancer cells in patients undergoing real-time immunosuppressive radiation and chemical treatments for cancer.[126] As a result of one set of these experiments, Southam and his colleagues expressed the hope that "the relation of host defenses to the course of human cancer might be studied fruitfully in patients with immunologic disorders."[127]

Could the AIDS epidemic, which is providing medical researchers with millions of cancer patients afflicted with useful "immunologic disorders," have been deliberately caused by cancer researchers following in Southam's footsteps—but using a more sophisticated procedure to deliberately *induce* immunosuppression? Did this sophisticated procedure consist of unleashing the animal immunosuppressive viruses (which had been adapted for human growth in the late 1970s) on human populations as a follow-up to Southam's experiments on a global scale?

The intentional use of human immunosuppressive viruses would have powerful experimental benefits. It would allow real-time modulation of the human immune system that would be very beneficial to cancer researchers. Such "active" immunosuppression would allow researchers to conduct experiments with human cancer susceptibility similar to those conducted by Southam—but these experiments would in fact be far more powerful. Instead of having to find patients with naturally occurring immune disorders, such disorders could be custom-produced on-demand for experiments designed to controllably increase human susceptibility to cancer under the watchful eyes of medical researchers (such cancers might result from natural exposure to carcinogenic agents or through injections of such agents). Such a procedure would allow researchers to watch cancer grow in thousands of subjects from its earliest and most critical stages in those predisposed to develop the disease.[128]

The use of such an experimental procedure might indeed explain the fact that the human AIDS virus has remarkable similarities to animal immunosuppressive viruses such as SIV (simian immunodeficiency virus) and BIV (bovine immunodeficiency virus). Readers skeptical of this theory may find it interesting that immunosuppressive cattle viruses such as bovine-visna virus[129] and immunosuppressive simian viruses such as the Mason Pfizer Monkey Virus (MPMV)[130] were being grown in human cell cultures[131] just prior to the AIDS epidemic.

The Mason Pfizer Monkey Virus causes a wasting disease in monkeys followed by infection with opportunistic diseases. While this virus is not the same SIV which is thought to have caused HIV, the effects of this virus in monkeys are similar to the effect of human infection with HIV.[132] This virus has been available to researchers since at least 1970–as were others.[133]

Readers who are skeptical that government-financed cancer researchers would inject human subjects with live viruses to modulate their immune systems so that changes in deliberately induced cancers could be measured should recall the set of experiments conducted by Southam. In them (partly sponsored by the U.S. Department of the Army), human subjects were exposed to various live viruses in combination with implants of human cancer cells. As Southam reported, he injected these viruses (West Nile[134], Mengo and Semliki Forest viruses) "shortly before, during, or after the implant studies."[135] (The co-injection of these viral "therapeutic agents" also allowed Southam to measure the anti-body response of the human subjects to the viruses so that it could be correlated with the response to the cancer implants.)

Those who are still skeptical that cancer researchers would inject human subjects undergoing immunosuppressive treatments with cancer-causing animal viruses should be aware of another group of precedent-setting experiments. In these experiments, which were based on and inspired by Southam's earlier studies,[136] patients of varying immune system health *were injected with cancer-causing monkey viruses to determine whether such viruses were capable of*

31

causing human cancer.[137] More precisely, naturally immunosuppressed human subjects and subjects who were being given immunosuppressive treatments for cancer were systematically injected with a dazzling array of mixtures of different types of human cells (including cancer cells) *and* animal cancer viruses, such as the simian cancer virus SV40. This experiment was similar to an experiment Southam conducted by exposing mice to immunosuppressive treatments and then injecting them with cancer transplants to measure how this affected cancer growth.[138] The researchers even got to use one of the same immunosuppressive treatments (an immunosuppressive chemical known as Cytoxan) in human transplant studies[139] that Southam used in cancer transplant studies in mice.[140]

In a 20-page paper in the *Journal of the National Cancer Institute*, researchers published table after table of the results of their attempts to induce tumors in human subjects (cancer patients) of various ages and in various disease states.[141] As occurred in the earlier forms of transplantable cancer experiments, tumors eventually grew in the immunosuppressed human patients as a result of these monkey cancer virus injections. (Experiments similar to these were conducted in monkeys in which immunosuppression and infection with the SV40 virus were studied to determine the cancer-causing potential of SV40.[142])

The researchers described which of the many mixtures of human cells and monkey cancer viruses they used resulted in tumor formation in their human victims. They began by using separate injections of human cancer cells and animal cancer viruses in different regions of the same subject's body. Because initially only the human cancer cell implants resulted in tumors, while the SV40 implants did not, researchers began to systematically investigate the mechanism by which the monkey virus SV40 could be made to cause human tumors. Experimental parameters investigated included: the length of time the SV40 was cultured in human cells, the type of human cancer cells the SV40 cancer virus was cultured with, the length of time the recipient subject had been on immunosuppressive drugs and the dose of cancer virus cells injected.

The experimentation with human subjects and the human cell/monkey cancer virus cultures eventually paid off. Researchers found that by using the right mixture of human cancer cells and the SV40 virus (cultured for the proper length of time and given in sufficient quantities), the SV40 monkey cancer virus could not only reproducibly cause tumors (referred to as "nodules") in human subjects, but could also be retrieved in cells removed from induced cancer growths. [143]

As the authors summarized:

> The formation of nodules after ...implantation of cells from simian virus 40 (SV40) transformed human tissue culture could be correlated with the stages of the transformation process, number of cells implanted, and possibly the presence of infectious virus in the implants.

While initially the researchers had more difficulty inducing human tumors with the SV40 virus than they did with just human cancer cells (such as HeLa cancer cells), eventually they found the SV40 monkey virus, when mixed and cultured properly, could produce human tumors (characterized as sarcomas) with comparable ease:

> Judging by the results of homologous implantation, HeLa cells and late passage, virus-free SV40-transformed cells had a comparable neoplastic potential. Histologically, nodules produced by SV40-transformed human cells were sarcomas.

In yet another series of experiments, both human cancer patients and test monkeys were injected with a monkey tumor virus known as the Yaba virus. After these virus injections, the researchers observed that, "The humans developed lesions quite similar to those of the monkeys" and, that "inoculation of virus produces only local tumors in the monkey and human."[144]

The unethical nature of these experiments is compounded by the fact that the researchers used human beings as walking tissue cultures for the monkey tumor virus they were studying—alternately inducing human tumors through injection of the monkey virus, removing tissue from the induced tumors, reinjecting the virus removed from the human tumors induced and, finally, inducing more tumors in other human subjects with the transplanted and processed virus.[145] The authors described this procedure as follows:

> A cell-free filtrate of a monkey tumor was injected into three sites on the left forearm, and

a tumor suspension into three sites on the right forearm of Patients 1, 2, and 3. Tumors developed at all sites. A single site was excised from the left forearm of Patient 2 at 17 days and from Patient 3 at 10 days. A suspension of each of these tumors was then injected into patient 5. ...Tumors developed at both sites; one site was excised at 10 days, and a suspension was injected into Patient 3. ... By this method, replication of the virus in the human was established.

Very similar procedures were used in experiments with mice to create the first proven mouse cancer viruses. Additionally, similar procedures were used in the concentration camps of Nazi Germany during medical experiments that will be described later.

* * *

In animal research with cancer viruses, researchers followed up their experiments with cancer virus injections with injections of immunosuppressive viruses. This was done to gain a more thorough understanding of how cancer viruses induced cancer as well as to make cancer grow more predictably. Knowledge of these experiments raises several questions with respect to AIDS:

- Did cancer researchers inject human subjects with animal immunosuppressive viruses in follow-up experiments to those in which they injected human subjects with numerous animal cancer and tumor viruses?

- Did such a process allow researchers to replicate in human populations the documented experimental procedure used extensively in animal immunosuppressive cancer research to prove the immunodeficiency and viral theory of cancer causation?
- Is this why the AIDS epidemic is proving so useful to cancer researchers investigating the viral causes of and potential vaccines for human cancers?

Indeed, if researchers were willing to cause cancer in human subjects by using monkey cancer viruses such as SV40, might they not have used monkey immunosuppressive viruses similar to MPMV in similar follow-up experiments? Before the AIDS epidemic began in humans, such viruses, which had been isolated as far back as 1970,[146] were known to cause disease states in monkeys that are similar to the wasting effects and immunodeficiency states that result from HIV infection in humans.[147] Additionally, the immunosuppressive MPMV virus was not only grown in an array of different human cells (including cancer cells)[148] prior to the AIDS epidemic, but also was combined with monkey cancer viruses such as SV40[149] (which had already been injected in human subjects) and simian sarcoma virus[150] and grown in human cell cultures prior to AIDS in humans. The effects on human immune system cells of similar viruses derived from human cancers were also systematically studied in the 1970s and 80s.[151]

The Benefits of the AIDS Epidemic

> The AIDS-malignancies have provided insights into the pathogenesis of neoplastic disease in general *and into strategies for further therapeutic intervention.* In the future, it is hoped that survival may be prolonged in affected patients *and that these disorders may be prevented.*[152] [emphasis added]

Although it does not constitute proof of deliberate, premeditated experimentation, it is highly suggestive that dramatic progress in human cancer research, similar to that made in animal cancer research using immunosuppressive techniques, is being made, and will most likely continue to be made, as a result of the immunosuppressive HIV epidemic.

Specifically, the alleged "AIDS experiment" that has resulted in greatly increased rates of cancers in immunosuppressed human subjects will most likely result in the stunning fulfillment of the three major goals of the viral cancer research establishment noted above:

- Proving that human cancer could be caused by viruses;
- Proving that a faulty immune system increased susceptibility to these viruses;
- Demonstrating that vaccines against such cancer viruses could be created by boosting the human immune system.

The AIDS virus has allowed cancer researchers to make a major breakthrough—providing long-awaited proof[153] that viruses cause sarcoma in humans. Headlines in the *New York Times* have announced that such viruses have been isolated from AIDS patients suffering from the most prominent form of AIDS-related cancer called Kaposi's sarcoma.[154] Although it is not known for sure that the virus is totally responsible for the growth of Kaposi's sarcoma in AIDS victims, this line of research is extremely encouraging to those studying the viral causes of human cancers. Lawrence Altman in the *New York Times* recently predicted: "Ultimately, the new findings about the Kaposi's sarcoma virus could help unravel many unknowns about how viruses cause cancers."

This line of research, which, at long-last, correlated a herpes virus to the growth of Kaposi's sarcoma in human subjects,[155] encouraged another group of researchers to look for other forms of cancer that might be caused by this same virus. These researchers have recently announced another major breakthrough in viral cancer research—finding a link between this same virus and a common form of blood cancer known as multiple myeloma, the second most prevalent form of blood cancer in the U.S.[156]

In addition to meeting the long-sought goal of demonstrating a viral cause of human cancer, the AIDS epidemic may also assist in meeting the other two main goals of the cancer virus research community—verifying the existence of a natural immunity to cancer and exploiting this immunity to create cancer vaccines.

By monitoring the development of AIDS-related cancers in HIV victims as their immune systems deteriorate, researchers have concluded that it is indeed *the destruction of a natural immunity to cancer that allows cancer growth to proliferate.* This view was stated by one researcher (with respect to AIDS-related cancers suspected of being caused by the Epstein Barr virus) as follows:

> Patients with ... acquired immunodeficiency disorders are vulnerable to a broad spectrum of opportunistic infectious diseases, but a narrow spectrum of malignancies. *These malignancies ... are likely due to failure of immune surveillance to recognize virally transformed target cells.* The evidence for this hypothesis is substantial regarding Epstein-Barr virus-induced lymphoproliferative lesions in immunodeficient patients.[157] [emphasis added]

Other researchers have invoked this "immune surveillance" concept with respect to Kaposi's sarcoma, a form of cancer that frequently afflicts AIDS patients. These researchers have noted that the severity of Kaposi's sarcoma in AIDS patients is often proportional to the degree of immune system damage, thus lending credence to the theory that a healthy individual's immune system is able to prevent the disease even when exposed to Kaposi's sarcoma agents:

> It now seems likely that there are symptom-free carriers of the Kaposi agent and that *an individual's immune status determines the clinical manifestations of disease–the more intense the immunosuppression, the more disseminated and rapidly growing are the Kaposi lesions and the more aggressive is the disease.*[158] [emphasis added]

Thus, according to numerous researchers, the AIDS virus is playing a significant role in identifying not only the viruses that cause AIDS-related cancers but also the purported natural immune system mechanisms capable of preventing cancer. Such direct proof that immunosurveillance exists for cancer in humans has been actively sought for decades.

Additionally, the AIDS epidemic is providing researchers with the ability to study cancer growth in humans not only as a function of immune system destruction and stimulation, but also as a function of environmental factors. As one group of researchers summarized with respect to the main form of cancer (Kaposi's sarcoma or KS) caused by HIV:

> The appearance of the AIDS epidemic has offered the opportunity to investigate the relationship between immune stimulation and immune dysregulation, lifestyle factors and KS tumour cell proliferation.[159]

Similar benefits were derived from animal experiments using manufactured immunosuppressive viruses in deliberate experimentation.

The importance of AIDS-related cancers to the cancer research community, as a means of identifying cancer causes in general, was admitted at the very earliest stages of the epidemic. For example, 20 years ago, in 1981, Altman wrote in the *New York Times* about the potential benefits to cancer research in general due to the AIDS-related Kaposi's sarcoma epidemic:

> The sudden appearance of the cancer, called Kaposi's sarcoma, has prompted *a medical investigation that experts say could have as much scientific as public health importance because of what it may teach about determining the causes of more common types of cancer.*[160] [emphasis added]

Since AIDS gives invaluable insight into the causes of cancer (both the viruses and the immune system defects), the AIDS epidemic will therefore likely play a critical role in aiding the development of strategies for cancer prevention. This optimistic view was summarized in the *New York Times*, as follows:

> If scientists can identify such protective mechanisms and other viruses that help produce H.I.V.-related tumors, then they can target them in developing new strategies to prevent Burkitt's and other cancers. For example, several scientists reported using such an approach in treating Epstein-Barr-related lymphomas.[161]

On to the achievement of the final goal...

Researchers studying the development of cancers in immunosuppressed AIDS patients have become convinced that, not only do cancer viruses cause human cancer, and that AIDS-related immune system damage destroys a suspected *natural ability* to reject cancer viruses in human patients, but also that a means of cancer prevention including vaccination will result from the knowledge gained in fighting the

AIDS/cancer epidemic. Wrote one researcher studying AIDS-induced tumors or "neoplasms":

> The occurrence of these neoplasms offers an opportunity to study the role of viruses and immunodeficiency in development of these tumors. Also, the pathogenic mechanisms leading to specific malignancies can be elucidated. *This information ought to guide development of strategies for prevention of virally determined cancers.*[162] [emphasis added]

Other authors in the *European Journal of Cancer* summarized the benefits of AIDS to cancer research in the following manner:

> As disastrous as the spread of HIV is, the insights that the AIDS epidemic provides into the causes of cancer *may ultimately lead to new and successful approaches to cancer prevention.*[163] [emphasis added]

Indeed, the AIDS epidemic is providing a near ideal research vehicle for proving theories about cancer causation that were popular shortly before the epidemic broke out. In 1972, the *Proceedings of the National Academy of Sciences* published numerous articles specifically speculating not only on the relationship between immunodeficiency[164] and viruses[165] in cancer formation, but also on the relationship between herpes viruses and cancers.[166] AIDS has apparently shown that immunodeficiencies can be a major contributor to cancer due to viruses and that one of the main forms of cancer due to such immunodeficiencies—Kaposi's sarcoma—is due to a herpes virus.

It should be clear that the HIV epidemic is providing cancer researchers with extensive knowledge of human cancer viruses and the immune system reactions to them. This knowledge will certainly assist in the development of human cancer vaccines. *But HIV itself may even be used in such vaccines if recent animal research is applicable to human cancer prevention.* Recent cancer experiments with HIV in animals have shown that the virus can be used not only to cause cancer but to inhibit its growth in the form of cancer vaccines!

By using components of HIV in experimental vaccines against tumors (which were induced by modified forms of HIV), researchers have reportedly dissected the role of CD4 and CD8 T-cells in tumor prevention through immunosurveillance. As one group of scientists reported, " … this model has allowed us to begin to dissect some of the mechanisms mediating and regulating tumor immunosurveillance." The researchers who conducted this experiment optimistically noted that this line of experimentation with HIV "may provide a successful concerted approach to cancer immunotherapy."

I suggest that this same goal in human cancer research (dissecting the role of T-cells in human cancer immunotherapy) is exactly why HIV was created and unleashed in human populations. However, in the human case, the HIV virus was likely an animal immunosuppressive virus modified for human growth to destroy subsets of the T-cell population to controllably increase cancer susceptibility for cancer vaccine research. In the case just cited, the *human* immunosuppressive virus was modified for animal growth and used to cause cancer and then to stimulate the immune system to inhibit cancer in the form of a vaccine.[167] Whether HIV will be used directly as a cancer vaccine in humans in a similar manner remains to be seen. However, as discussed below, the use of HIV in genetic therapy in humans looks promising.

Cancer researchers are not the only ones who are benefiting from the medical knowledge gained in the fight against AIDS. The entire medical research community stands to reap tremendously useful knowledge from the AIDS catastrophe. As several knowledgeable authors summarized in the medical literature:

> Furthermore, an unforeseen dividend for HIV research is the unraveling of the rich, intricate pathways of gene regulation utilized by the virus, which may well illuminate novel, fundamental cellular processes. *The understanding of basic biology that we gain from the studies of HIV may be one major legacy of this epidemic to medical science.*[168] [emphasis added]

The knowledge gained in the fight against AIDS and cancer will also directly benefit the pharmaceuticals companies developing AIDS diagnostic, therapeutic and preventive procedures as well as companies developing human cancer vaccines.

But HIV may have much more far-reaching medical uses than cancer vaccines—as stunning as that achievement might be.

Indeed, HIV has the potential to be a very useful virus with broad biomedical applications. Amazingly enough, researchers have begun using the HIV virus itself as a viral "vector" for the controversial line of medicine known as gene therapy—at least in the laboratory. By deleting certain genes in the deadly AIDS virus, researchers have been able to exploit its unique infectious properties while eliminating its harmful capacity. As summarized by Andrew Pollack in the *New York Times*:

> In a bold but potentially frightening effort to turn one of the world's most virulent killers into a cure, scientists and biotechnology companies are trying to tame the AIDS virus and harness it to treat disease. The scientists say they have stripped the human immunodeficiency virus of its ability to cause disease, while leaving intact its ability to infect human cells. Such a crippled virus, they say, could be used to deliver genes in to human cells for gene therapy.

As a result of laboratory tests, the subfamily of viruses to which HIV belongs is thought to be one of those most suited for the emerging technology of genetic therapy. This type of virus, the lentivirus, seems to have infectious properties which render it superior to other viruses for the insertion of genes in human DNA. This includes the DNA of nondividing cells, which pose a barrier to other types of viral vectors. As noted by Pollack in the *Times*:

> H.I.V., on the other hand, is both cunning at evading the body's immune defenses and can carry large genes. Most important, it is one of a small class of viruses, known as lentiviruses, that can incorporate genes into the chromosomes even of nondividing cells.[169]

This convenient infectious property, together with its carrying capacity, makes HIV one of the more promising ones for use in human clinical gene therapy trials.

* * *

It should be evident that the AIDS epidemic is proving fantastically beneficial to cancer researchers—the same group that created the first immunosuppressive viruses as a weapon in the war on cancer long before the Human Immunosuppressive Virus began infecting human populations. Is this just the result of good fortune on the part of the cancer scientists or did some of them play more of an active role in acquiring such human research models and lucrative data than they have let on? Certainly, the researchers aren't going to talk, though others have suggested what they may be doing[170] to make AIDS even more deadly and infective than it already is.[171] However, Altman, a *New York Times* journalist who has been chronicling the progression of AIDS and its positive impact on cancer research for some time, made the following observation with regard to the relation of the HIV epidemic and the government's war on cancer:

> Because H.I.V. suppresses the immune system and most AIDS-related cancers are strongly associated with viruses, *scientists saw in the tragedy of the AIDS epidemic an extraordinary opportunity to study the interplay of viruses, an impaired immune system and the development of cancer. In a way, AIDS research was an extension of the war on cancer that the Government declared in 1971.*[172] [emphasis added]

If the hypothesis of this study is true, and AIDS was created as a tool in the war on cancer (just as MAIDS and FAIDS were), Altman may have revealed more than he realized in this illuminating comment.

Why Were Homosexuals Targeted?

Readers may naturally wonder why homosexuals would have been chosen in the alleged cancer experiment. There may be a simple answer to this question. Recall that cancer researchers were extremely interested in determining whether viruses could cause human cancer. One reason why there was such intense interest in this subject was that if such viruses were causing human cancer, then it might be possible to manipulate these viruses, or similar viruses,[173] into serving as vaccines against cancer—just as the polio virus had been manipulated to serve as a vaccine against polio.[174] As Southam once observed: "If and when a causative virus of human cancers is found, it may provide a source of antigen for cancer prophylaxis, but this is merely a hope for the future."[175]

Homosexuals were known to be already disproportionately infected with viruses (for example, hepatitis and cytomegalovirus) that were thought to be capable of inducing cancer.[176] By monitoring cancer rates in otherwise healthy homosexuals (as a control group) known to be infected with these viruses, and then monitoring cancer rates in this same group after it was ravaged by immunosuppression, researchers are able to correlate both the degree of immunosuppression and the degree of viral infection in this group with cancer.[177] Thus, the experiments in mice in which researchers injected both cancer viruses and immunosuppressive viruses might be replicated in human populations merely through the injection of immunosuppressive viruses, if populations already infected with cancer viruses were chosen for the experiment.[178]

Viruses subsequently proved to be capable of causing cancer *only after immunosuppression took effect* in these studies might be the subject of follow-up experiments in which these viruses would be manipulated as potential cancer vaccines.

Summary
Numerous precedents have been reviewed that make the radical theory proposed here seem more plausible. These precedents include the exploitation of immunosuppression to induce human cancer growth through decades of systematic injections of human guinea pigs with cancer cells and cancer-causing monkey and tumor viruses.[179] The modification of the experimental procedure used in these experiments to include injections of animal *immunosuppressive* viruses (which existed long before AIDS broke out in human populations), along with the implementation of

such a procedure on an international scale,[180] could very well explain the *form* of the international epidemic of HIV.

BIOLOGICAL TESTING INVOLVING HUMAN SUBJECTS BY THE DEPARTMENT OF DEFENSE, 1977

HEARINGS

BEFORE THE

SUBCOMMITTEE ON
HEALTH AND SCIENTIFIC RESEARCH

OF THE

COMMITTEE ON HUMAN RESOURCES
UNITED STATES SENATE

NINETY-FIFTH CONGRESS

FIRST SESSION

ON

EXAMINATION OF SERIOUS DEFICIENCIES IN THE DEFENSE
DEPARTMENT'S EFFORTS TO PROTECT THE HUMAN SUBJECTS
OF DRUG RESEARCH

MARCH 8 AND MAY 23, 1977

Printed for the use of the Committee on Human Resources

U.S. GOVERNMENT PRINTING OFFICE
WASHINGTON : 1977

97-857 O

Congress investigates military's tests on human subjects.

HUMAN DRUG TESTING BY THE CIA, 1977

DEPOSITORY 594

HEARINGS

FEB 15 1978

BEFORE THE

SUBCOMMITTEE ON
HEALTH AND SCIENTIFIC RESEARCH

OF THE

COMMITTEE ON HUMAN RESOURCES
UNITED STATES SENATE

NINETY-FIFTH CONGRESS

FIRST SESSION

ON

S. 1893

TO AMEND THE PUBLIC HEALTH SERVICE ACT TO ESTABLISH
THE PRESIDENT'S COMMISSION FOR THE PROTECTION OF
HUMAN SUBJECTS OF BIOMEDICAL AND BEHAVIORAL RE-
SEARCH, AND FOR OTHER PURPOSES

SEPTEMBER 20 AND 21, 1977

❀

Printed for the use of the Committee on Human Resources

U.S. GOVERNMENT PRINTING OFFICE
WASHINGTON : 1977

Congress investigates CIA's drug tests on human subjects.

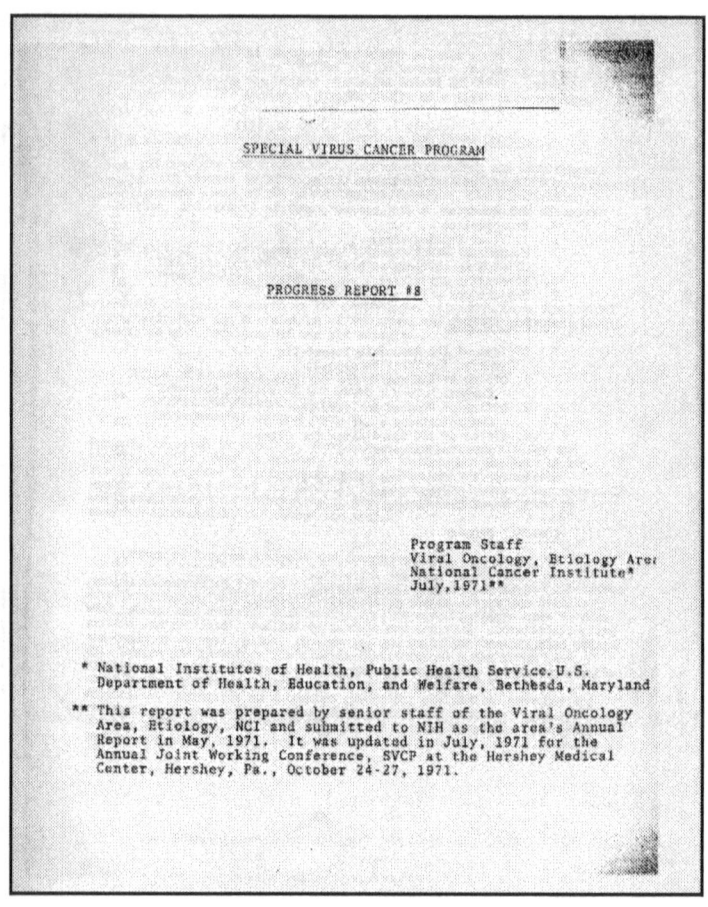

1971 National Cancer Institute Document: *Report #8 of the Special Virus Cancer Program* detailing crash project in 1970s to isolate and manufacture human and animal cancer viruses to develop human cancer vaccines.

AIDS: The "Perfect" Disease

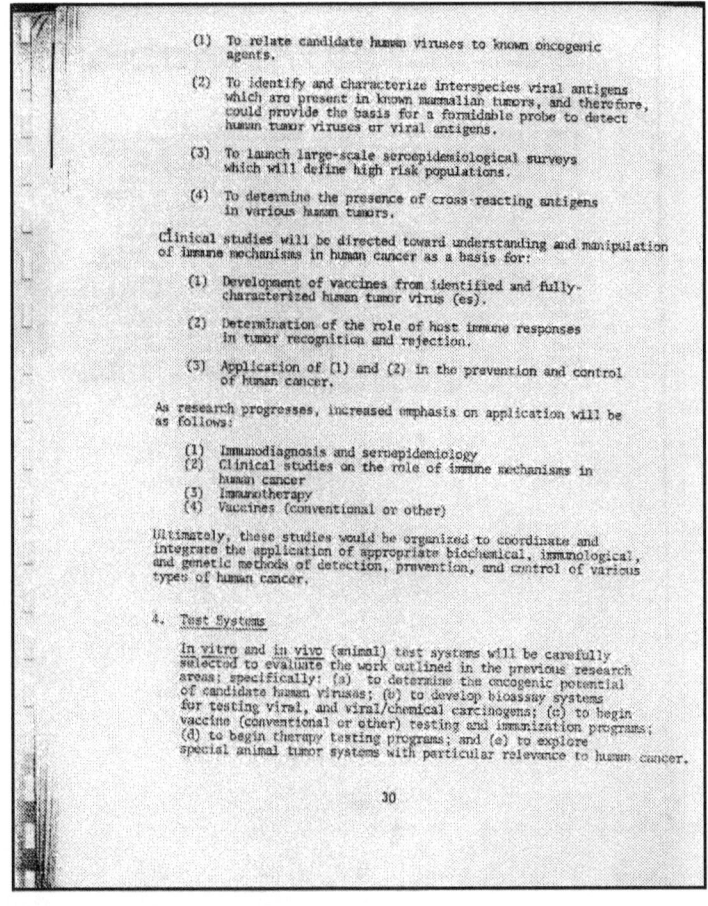

(1) To relate candidate human viruses to known oncogenic agents.

(2) To identify and characterize interspecies viral antigens which are present in known mammalian tumors, and therefore, could provide the basis for a formidable probe to detect human tumor viruses or viral antigens.

(3) To launch large-scale seroepidemiological surveys which will define high risk populations.

(4) To determine the presence of cross-reacting antigens in various human tumors.

Clinical studies will be directed toward understanding and manipulation of immune mechanisms in human cancer as a basis for:

(1) Development of vaccines from identified and fully-characterized human tumor virus (es).

(2) Determination of the role of host immune responses in tumor recognition and rejection.

(3) Application of (1) and (2) in the prevention and control of human cancer.

As research progresses, increased emphasis on application will be as follows:

(1) Immunodiagnosis and seroepidemiology
(2) Clinical studies on the role of immune mechanisms in human cancer
(3) Immunotherapy
(4) Vaccines (conventional or other)

Ultimately, these studies would be organized to coordinate and integrate the application of appropriate biochemical, immunological, and genetic methods of detection, prevention, and control of various types of human cancer.

4. Test Systems

In vitro and in vivo (animal) test systems will be carefully selected to evaluate the work outlined in the previous research areas; specifically: (a) to determine the oncogenic potential of candidate human viruses; (b) to develop bioassay systems for testing viral, and viral/chemical carcinogens; (c) to begin vaccine (conventional or other) testing and immunization programs; (d) to begin therapy testing programs; and (e) to explore special animal tumor systems with particular relevance to human cancer.

30

Special Virus Cancer Program goals outlined for human cancer vaccine effort: Isolate and produce human cancer viruses ("determine the oncogenic potential of candidate human viruses"); Verify an immune response to these viruses ("Determination of the role of host immune responses in tumor recognition and rejection;"); Develop cancer virus vaccines ("development of vaccines from identified and fully characterized human tumor virus").

AIDS is providing the perfect vehicle for the fulfillment of these lofty goals, the first two of which have already been achieved. HIV is also being used in animal studies to achieve the third (see text).

53

> these cell lines have revealed additional evidence consistent with presence in the cells of an RNA tumor virus: the presence of the RNA-dependent DNA polymerase, the interspecies antigen.
>
> Breast cancer occurs in about 4 to 5% of American women. It is the most prevalent and responsible for more deaths than any other type of cancer, not only in American women but also among women of several other countries. Because breast cancer occurs 2 or 3 times more frequently in some families than in others it is strikingly similar to observations made on breast cancer of different populations of mice. These animal studies led to unequivocal evidence of the association of a virus and the demonstration that an infectious form of it is transmitted through milk. One of the major objectives of the SVCP is now the determination whether an agent similar to that of mice is responsible for the unusually high incidence of breast cancer in certain human populations.
>
> ### Herpes-type Viruses
>
> A type of virus associated with some forms of chronic leukemia, lymphoma, and postnasal carcinoma is the herpes-type virus (HTV), similar in size and shape but not identical to other known herpesviruses. Unlike these Type C particles, HTV grows well in the laboratory and fairly large quantities of purified and concentrated HTV can be recovered for study. One of the most active areas of viral oncology is that concerned with definitive characterization of the HTV.
>
> Considerable interest has developed in the herpes group of viruses as cancer-causing agents in animals and man. Herpes-type viruses have been shown to induce kidney carcinomas of the frog and to be causally related to lymphoproliferative diseases in chickens, monkeys, marmosets and rabbits. Projects within the Program have focused on the significance of the Epstein-Barr virus (EBV) from Burkitt's lymphoma and postnasal carcinoma and Herpesvirus hominus type 2 (HSV-2) from cervical carcinoma.
>
> Seroepidemiological studies on the relationship of EBV infection to nasopharyngeal cancer are being conducted through the International Agency for Research on Cancer. A study in the West Nile District of Uganda to determine the feasibility of further studies on EBV in relation to Burkitt's tumor is nearing completion. Other studies also suggest an association between infection by HSV-2 and cervical carcinoma. Results of a study made in Texas showed the presence of serum antibodies to this virus in about 45% of cases of invasive cervical carcinoma in comparison to 22% in controls. Recent findings in Colombia showed a much higher incidence of antibody in the control population selected, approximating the incidence in the tumor-bearing group. At present, insufficient data is available to conclude that this virus is implicated in this cancer.
>
> EBV infection has been associated with the development of infectious mononucleosis in young adults, a disease with the attributes of a self-limiting leukemia. The generally high levels of antibodies to EBV in patients
>
> 25

Special Virus Cancer Program Report #8 identified Herpes viruses for extensive study in humans. According to this report Herpes-type virus (HTV) "grows well in the laboratory and fairly large quantities of purified and concentrated HTV can be recovered for study." Researchers lamented: "At present, insufficient data is available to conclude that this virus (Epstein-Barr virus) is implicated in this cancer." In remarkable breakthroughs, AIDS is providing volumes of long-sought data implicating EBV and other herpes viruses in human cancer due to infection with HIV. (Prior to AIDS, EBV from human cancers had already been isolated and injected in rats to cause cancer.) Were HIV and HTV used in subsequent studies recommended in the report ("clinical studies will be directed toward understanding and manipulation of immune mechanisms in human cancer")?

NATIONAL SECURITY COUNCIL
WASHINGTON, D.C. 20506

UNCLASSIFIED

April 24, 1974

National Security Study Memorandum 200

TO:
    The Secretary of Defense
    The Secretary of Agriculture
    The Director of Central Intelligence
    The Deputy Secretary of State
    Administrator, Agency for International Development

SUBJECT:
    Implications of Worldwide Population Growth for U.S.
    Security and Overseas Interests

The President has directed a study of the impact of world population growth on U.S. security and overseas interests. The study should look forward at least until the year 2000, and use several alternative reasonable projections of population growth.

In terms of each projection, the study should assess:

-- the corresponding pace of development, especially in poorer countries;

-- the demand for US exports, especially of food, and the trade problems the US may face arising from competition for resources; and

-- the likelihood that population growth or imbalances will produce disruptive foreign policies and international instability.

The study should focus on the international political and economic implications of population growth rather than its ecological, sociological or other aspects.

The study should then offer possible courses of action for the United States in dealing with population matters abroad, particularly in developing countries, with special attention to these questions:

-- What, if any, new initiatives by the United States are needed to focus international attention on the population problem?

-- Can technological innovations or development reduce growth or ameliorate its effects?

UNCLASSIFIED

Declassified on July 3, 1989
by the National Security Council,
under provisions of E.O. 12065.

Declassified National Security Council study outlining aggressive U.S. global depopulation plans for Third World.

Jerry Leonard

NATIONAL SECURITY COUNCIL
WASHINGTON, D.C. 20506

 (GDS)

November 26, 1975

National Security Decision Memorandum 314

TO: The Secretary of State
        The Secretary of the Treasury
        The Secretary of Defense
        The Secretary of Agriculture
        The Secretary of Health, Education and Welfare
        The Administrator, Agency for International Development

SUBJECT: Implications of Worldwide Population Growth for United
          States Security and Overseas Interests

The President has reviewed the interagency response to NSSM 200 and the covering memorandum from the Chairman of the NSC Under Secretaries Committee   He believes that United States leadership is essential to combat population growth, to implement the World Population Plan of Action and to advance United States security and overseas interests.   The President endorses the policy recommendations contained in the Executive Summary of the NSSM 200 response, with the following observations and exceptions:

AID Programs

Care must be taken that our AID program efforts are not so diffuse as to have little impact upon those countries contributing the largest growth in population, and where reductions in fertility are most needed for economic and social progress.

Research and Evaluation

An examination should be undertaken of the effectiveness of population control programs in countries at all levels of development, but with

 (GDS)

Declassified/Released on _____ F84-135
under provisions of E.O. 12356
By R. Reger, National Security Council

NSC memo that resulted in National Security Council being put in charge of U.S. population efforts overseas.

56

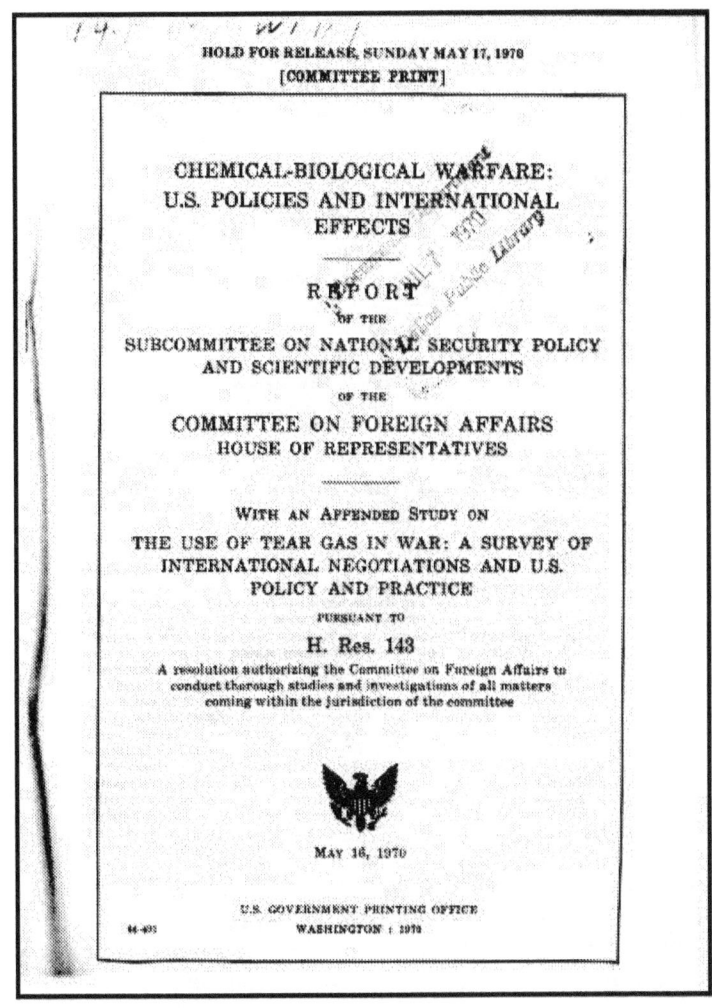

1970 congressional investigation of U.S. chemical-biological warfare policy:

"... on the immediate horizon are modern developments in molecular genetics which could result in manmade viruses for which there would be no natural immunities and against which no reasonable defense could be mounted."

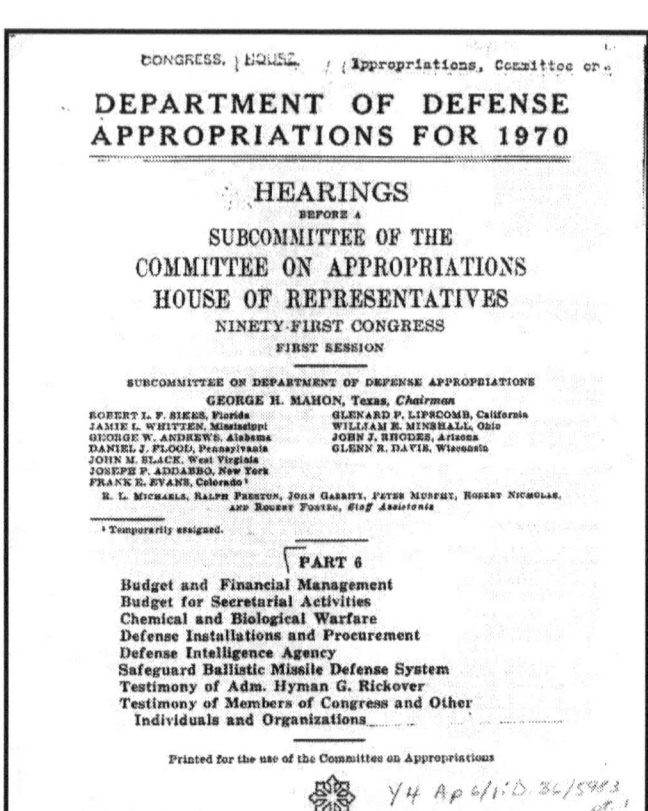

CONGRESS. | HOUSE. / {Appropriations, Committee or..

DEPARTMENT OF DEFENSE
APPROPRIATIONS FOR 1970

HEARINGS
BEFORE A
SUBCOMMITTEE OF THE
COMMITTEE ON APPROPRIATIONS
HOUSE OF REPRESENTATIVES
NINETY-FIRST CONGRESS
FIRST SESSION

SUBCOMMITTEE ON DEPARTMENT OF DEFENSE APPROPRIATIONS
GEORGE H. MAHON, Texas, *Chairman*

ROBERT L. F. SIKES, Florida   GLENARD P. LIPSCOMB, California
JAMIE L. WHITTEN, Mississippi   WILLIAM E. MINSHALL, Ohio
GEORGE W. ANDREWS, Alabama   JOHN J. RHODES, Arizona
DANIEL J. FLOOD, Pennsylvania   GLENN R. DAVIS, Wisconsin
JOHN M. SLACK, West Virginia
JOSEPH P. ADDABBO, New York
FRANK E. EVANS, Colorado¹

R. L. MICHAELS, RALPH PRESTON, JOHN GARRITY, PETER MURPHY, ROBERT NICHOLAS,
AND ROBERT FOSTER, *Staff Assistants*

¹ Temporarily assigned.

PART 6
Budget and Financial Management
Budget for Secretarial Activities
Chemical and Biological Warfare
Defense Installations and Procurement
Defense Intelligence Agency
Safeguard Ballistic Missile Defense System
Testimony of Adm. Hyman G. Rickover
Testimony of Members of Congress and Other
   Individuals and Organizations

Printed for the use of the Committee on Appropriations

Y 4 Ap 6/1:D 36/5983
pt. 1

1970 DOD appropriations hearings: "Within a period of 5 to 10 years, it would be possible to make a new infective microorganism which could differ in certain important aspects from any known disease-causing organisms. Most important of these is that it might be refractory to the immunological and therapeutic processes upon which we depend to maintain our relative freedom from infectious disease.... It is a highly controversial issue, and there are many who believe such research should not be undertaken lest it lead to yet another method of massive killing of large populations."

BIOMEDICAL AND BEHAVIORAL RESEARCH, 1975

JOINT HEARINGS

BEFORE THE

SUBCOMMITTEE ON HEALTH

OF THE

COMMITTEE ON
LABOR AND PUBLIC WELFARE

AND THE

SUBCOMMITTEE ON
ADMINISTRATIVE PRACTICE AND PROCEDURE

OF THE

COMMITTEE ON THE JUDICIARY
UNITED STATES SENATE

NINETY-FOURTH CONGRESS

FIRST SESSION

ON

HUMAN-USE EXPERIMENTATION PROGRAMS OF THE DEPART-
MENT OF DEFENSE AND CENTRAL INTELLIGENCE AGENCY

AND

S. 2515

TO AMEND THE PUBLIC HEALTH SERVICE ACT TO ESTABLISH
THE PRESIDENT'S COMMISSION FOR THE PROTECTION OF
HUMAN SUBJECTS INVOLVED IN BIOMEDICAL AND BE-
HAVIORAL RESEARCH, AND FOR OTHER PURPOSES

SEPTEMBER 10, 12; AND NOVEMBER 7, 1975

Printed for the use of the Committee on Labor and Public Welfare
and the Committee on the Judiciary

U.S. GOVERNMENT PRINTING OFFICE
70-098 O   WASHINGTON : 1976

1975 Senate investigation of CIA and DOD testing on human subjects; list of projects at army hospitals included "Evaluation and Study of Patients with Primary and Secondary Immunodeficiency Diseases."

The National Security Angle

In addition to the advancement of cancer research (including the likely development of cancer vaccines), a hidden benefit of the AIDS epidemic is the imminent fulfillment of long-standing U.S. "national security" goals. These goals are associated with the depopulation effect the epidemic will soon have (barring a medical breakthrough in curing AIDS) in the Third World. This effect will most likely meet many of the goals set forth by the U.S. National Security Council (NSC) in a comprehensive, classified population control study conducted in the early 1970s–shortly before the AIDS epidemic broke out. The extraordinary NSC study, entitled "Implications Of Worldwide Population Growth For U.S. Security And Overseas Interests," recommended an aggressive global depopulation effort as a means of maintaining access to Third World resources on behalf of U.S. corporations.

Recognizing that the United States was extremely dependent on foreign sources of natural resources, especially in the developing world,[181] the relationship between global access to resources and international population reduction (as a "stabilizing" influence) was bluntly summarized in the study as follows:

> "Whatever may be done to guard against interruptions of supply and to develop domestic alternatives, the U.S. economy will require large and increasing amounts of minerals from abroad, especially from less developed countries. That fact gives the U.S. enhanced interest in the political, economic, and social stability of the supplying countries. *Wherever a*

> *lessening of population pressures through reduced birth rates can increase the prospects for such stability, **population policy becomes relevant to resource supplies** and to the economic interests of the United States."* [emphasis added] [182]

The global locations of "needed" resources were mapped out in this study and specific country-by-country goals were set for massive, international U.S. depopulation efforts aimed at maintaining access to these resources.

Despite the efforts of the population control establishment at the time, the probability that the population control goals set by the U.S. government would be met in the Less Developed Countries (LDCs) appeared to be poor at best. This pessimistic viewpoint is evident in the NSC study. The fact that Third World population growth would at least double, and maybe triple—even if the advocated family planning programs were implemented—greatly troubled the NSC authors. As it was put in the NSC study:

> … short of Draconian measures there is no possibility that any LDC can stabilize its population at less than double its present size. For many, stabilization will not be short of three times their present size.[183]

Did the NSC resort to "Draconian" measures to "stabilize" the world's increasing population levels? If so, what sort of Draconian measures were available as options?

From the tone of the NSC study and statements from other government officials at the time, it is apparent that the international "population problem" was seen as a major threat to U.S. corporate interests.[184] The NSC, through the CIA, specialized in eliminating such national security threats using systematic state violence (using covert and overt wars) throughout the developing world whenever U.S. business interests were threatened (for example, in Vietnam and Guatemala).

As a direct result of this NSC study: *the Chairman of the National Security Council, the individual responsible for overseeing U.S. covert operations throughout the world, was given responsibility for implementing the stated international depopulation goals.*[185] In light of this development, it is curious that, barring a major medical breakthrough that provides a cheap and effective cure for AIDS,[186] these aggressive depopulation goals for certain areas of the Third World (which the NSC study authors doubted could be met in a timely manner by conventional methods) will likely be met with the help of the AIDS virus.[187]

For example, the NSC study stated "the goals proposed by the United States: For developing countries—replacement levels in two or three decades." The devastation produced by AIDS in parts of Africa has resulted in the predicted imminent achievement of this aggressive goal, which seemed hopeless when it was published. As was summarized in a CNN report: "Some of the countries most affected by AIDS epidemics are projected to have zero or near-zero population growth, because of the higher mortality rates combined with low projected fertility rates."[188]

If this trend continues, AIDS will provide a means of implementing both methods (increasing the death rate and decreasing the birth rate) for reducing population growth mentioned by the National Academy of Sciences:

> "Modern medicine and advances in nutrition have cut the death rates throughout the world, producing a fantastic population growth rate. The most frightening aspect of this growth rate is that if it continues, we will have 14 billion people or four times our present population by 2015. The National Academy of Sciences has said: *'Either the birth rate must come down or the death rate must go back up.'*"[189] [emphasis added]

Conveniently for the depopulation planners, AIDS is targeting the exact regions of the globe where, just prior to AIDS, most of the population increases were projected to take place. The Third World suffers 95% of worldwide AIDS deaths and is where the National Security Council predicted in 1974 that 90% of world population increases would occur by the year 2000.[190] (In an editorial, the *New York Times* also noted the striking disparity in the geography of the disease *treatment* versus the geography of the disease *distribution*: "Currently, some 95 percent of all the AIDS prevention money is being spent in the industrialized countries, while 95 percent of those infected live in the developing countries."[191])

The AIDS epidemic is especially pronounced in Africa, "the continent with the world's fastest-expanding population."[192] As reported by the Population Reference Bureau, "It seems quite likely that AIDS will alter the demographic prospects of some 20 to 30 [African] countries."[193] The report predicted a staggering 100 million AIDS-related deaths in Africa by the year 2025. Eastern and southern Africa, which have only 5% of the world's population, account for 60% of all AIDS deaths.[194] In the sub-Saharan regions of Africa, some nations such as Zimbabwe are projected to lose 25% of their populations to AIDS.[195]

If these trends continue, the increased death rate due to the AIDS virus itself may not only allow fulfillment of the "zero growth" goals of the population elite but may actually produce a negative population growth in some areas. (This need for negative growth has been justified recently under the banner of protecting the ecosystem.) This negative growth trend may already be realized in some countries in Africa such as Uganda, where scientists are predicting a negative population growth by the year 2002.[196] In fact, the AIDS virus may be so effective at reducing population growth in these regions that the U.S. government is already conceding that its major international initiative in "family planning" may no longer be necessary in some countries—except as a long-term means of maintaining low fertility rates. This reality was summarized in the *New York Times:* "Some officials in government already privately contend that family planning is not as necessary in Africa because AIDS will take care of the rapid growth in the population."[197]

It seems reasonable to speculate that the convenient depopulation of Third World regions as a result of the AIDS epidemic is not a happy coincidence for the national security establishment. It is more likely that this convenient effect was *designed* as the result of the implementation of a form of biowarfare[198] that was carried out under the pretext of a global cancer experiment.[199] Certainly the convenience of the effects of AIDS is not lost on the Africans. Sam Nujoma, the President of Namibia, which has adult HIV infection rates of approximately 20%, stated his belief that AIDS was a manufactured disease at a press conference in Geneva:

> We in Namibia are the sufferers of this dreadful disease. It is also a historical fact that HIV/AIDS is a man-made disease. It is not natural. States that produced chemical weapons to kill other nations are known, they are probably represented here, they know themselves too.[200]

Whether you believe that HIV was intentionally developed and implemented as a biowarfare weapon, the results of the virus in Africa certainly appear to be having the catastrophic effect of one. AIDS kills ten times as many people as wars in Africa. As the *New York Times* summarized:

> AIDS is now the leading killer in sub-Saharan Africa, a region where poverty and wars have already taken a heavy toll. In 1998, 200,000 people died as a result of armed conflicts in Africa, compared to about 2.2 million from AIDS.[201]

Precedent for Experimentation:

Many American citizens would no doubt recoil in horror at the thought of their government being involved in such cruel and devastating human experimentation. Yet the historical record is replete with precedents involving such large-scale and inhumane experimentation–especially when the national security excuse could be invoked to justify such measures. Witness the massive number of radiation experiments (thousands) that were covertly conducted on the U.S. population throughout the 1950s and 60s as an adjunct to radiation weapons development[202] or the infamous LSD experimentation conducted by the CIA on the public throughout the 1950s, 60s and 70s using the excuse that the Soviets were making significant advances in pharmacological mind control technology.

War Criminals and the U.S. Biowarfare Effort

Assuming the theory proposed above is accurate, who within the U.S. or international power structure might have been involved in the implementation of such an act of biological warfare under the guise of cancer experimentation?

Are there people working with the U.S. national security establishment with a history of committing such barbaric acts?

Just what people within the U.S. biowarfare effort had experience with massive, criminal human experimentation of this kind?

For starters, many Japanese biowarfare experts were recruited by the U.S. government immediately after World War II. These were the same people who had conducted experiments and massive field trials with chemical and biological warfare agents on the Chinese during World War II.[203] These biowarfare experts (working through the Japanese biological warfare research outfit called Unit 731) and war criminals were secretly pardoned by the US in trade for their tainted experimental data after the war.[204] In addition to Japanese war criminals, Nazi doctors with criminal pasts were secretly recruited after the war and put to work in the U.S. chemical warfare department.[205] (Other Nazi scientists with criminal pasts were brought into the U.S. to work on the space program.)

Before one rejects the thesis that Nazi or Japanese war criminals helped implement an American-backed global experiment involving immunosuppressive viruses through international humanitarian agencies such as the World Health Organization, realize that Nazi and Japanese "doctors" were installed in high-level post-war positions that would have allowed them to help implement such experiments. Nazi war figures have been found at the pinnacle of international humanitarian agencies such as the United Nations[206] and the World Medical Association,[207] and Japanese war figures found refuge in prestigious positions within the Japanese government, Japanese medical schools[208] and the international pharmaceuticals industry.[209]

Such well-placed individuals could have been useful to help implement any international biowarfare exercises or cancer experiments devised by their counterparts working with the U.S. national security establishment. Working together, Nazi and Japanese war criminals employed by the U.S. government and international agencies would have had highly relevant laboratory and field experience for implementing a large-scale experiment such as the AIDS situation. Nazi war criminals would have been able to apply the knowledge gained in the vaccine development experiments that they conducted on prisoners in the Nazi concentration camps. (These experiments involved manipulation of the immune system and injecting pathogens as a means of developing and testing future vaccines for German pharmaceutical companies.[210] Nazi concentration camp researchers also investigated means of transferring diseases from monkeys to man.) Similarly, the Japanese biowarfare criminals would have been able to apply their extensive expertise (gained on Chinese civilians during the war) on how to conduct very large-scale, international biowarfare-related "field trials" on entire populations.[211] (Shortly after the war, the U.S. government began conducting decades-long, large-scale biological warfare field trials in the U.S. According to Fort Detrick personnel "[c]ities were surreptitiously used as laboratories to test aerosolization and dispersal methods when simulants were released during covert experiments in New York City, San Francisco, and other sites between 1949 and 1968."[212])

Biological Warfare and Cancer Research

While a covert biological warfare program provided a pretext for employing an army of war personnel after World War II, cancer research provided a pretext for employing biowarfare experts after this biological warfare program was allegedly shut down.

As a result of congressional and international pressure, President Nixon decided to formally cancel the U.S. biological weapons research effort in 1969. Stocks of toxins were destroyed (although the CIA secretly maintained a biowarfare capability), President Nixon declared a national war on cancer and the Fort Detrick biowarfare research facility at Edgewood, Maryland, was converted to a cancer research facility in 1971. (This was not the first time that a biowarfare enterprise at Camp Detrick was converted to a civilian effort. After WWII, a pilot production effort aimed at manufacturing bombs filled with B anthracis was converted to a pharmaceutical lab.[213])

It has been postulated by some observers that Nixon's war on cancer was a convenient cover for the continuation of biowarfare research using civilian agencies. Government planners had already laid the groundwork for chemical and biological warfare research within civilian agencies.[214] The ease with which a research program in biological warfare could be conducted within civilian agencies was noted by an Army report as far back as 1946: "It is clear that the development of biological warfare could very well proceed in many countries, perhaps under the guise of legitimate medical or bacteriological research."[215] Dr. Joshua Lederberg stated in Congressional hearings that: "*BW defense is essentially the same as public health defense*. There are very few features–there are some, but they are not worth spending much time to discuss–that would distinguish the spread of a natural epidemic from the response to a concerted attack. *So one could argue that a large amount of public health work, is, in fact, defensively applicable to biological warfare*." [emphasis added][216]

The Defense Department still uses the defensive nature of its research (for example, work on vaccines to naturally occurring diseases) to justify extensive collaboration with the civilian sector. As was stated by one biowarfare researcher describing the extent of assistance from the Defense Department to the civilian research establishment:

> ... the broad scope of this research is possible because of an active program of DoD grants and contracts to universities, companies, and other institutes. These collaborations serve an important role in many of our research projects, providing the critical mass of scientific expertise required to manage a program with diverse technologies and requirements. The DoD extramural research program is a good example of our open research program and has led to some excellent scientific collaborations both in the United States and abroad.[217]

The war on cancer did allow the biological warfare research infrastructure to remain essentially intact. According to Richard Hatch writing in *Covert Action Information Bulletin*, the National Cancer Institute began funding the same researchers, universities and corporations in the war against cancer that had been funded during the biowarfare development effort.[218]

Many of the biowarfare researchers put to work on the war against cancer continued their work in biological warfare research. This research eventually included the production of huge quantities of cancer-causing viruses as well as the development of methods and delivery systems for the aerosol transmission of cancer viruses.[219] (This goal was accomplished when cancer researchers modified the cancer-causing AIDS virus to infect a new class of cells which would render it capable of being transmitted through the air. See section: The Benefits of the AIDS Epidemic.)

It was openly stated at the time of the conversion that the Fort Detrick facility would be used to produce cancer viruses. As noted by the *New York Times*: "Viruses and special biological materials will be produced in large quantities for use, not only at Fort Detrick, but also at other laboratories doing cancer research." The director of the cancer institute (Dr. Rauscher) told the *Times* that research at the facility would include research on viruses known to cause cancer in animals as well as on viruses suspected of having a role in human cancer.[220]

The fact that Fort Detrick had not abandoned its biowarfare activities despite the earlier pronouncements of abandoning germ warfare research by the U.S. government became obvious in 1982 when an article in the *New York Times* revealed that the researchers there were still engaged in what was labeled "defensive research" in germ warfare. This work was taking place under the cover of finding vaccines for potential biological warfare agents that could be used against the U.S. in an enemy attack. (Of course, in order to test vaccines for diseases likely to

71

be used for biowarfare, researchers had to first develop the diseases themselves in order to understand their potential harmful effects as well as the effectiveness of the relevant vaccine.[221])

The ability of the government to conduct large-scale and unethical weapons research under the guise of civilian research would hardly be unprecedented. A massive CIA crash program to develop mind control drugs and techniques, for example, was successfully operated for years in just this way. (The program was so successfully disguised and compartmentalized that many of the civilian researchers were not aware of the uses for which their research was intended.)

The most notorious program in this effort was project MKULTRA begun in 1953 which was described as "the principal CIA program involving the research and development of chemical and biological agents." It was "concerned with the research and development of chemical, biological, and radiological materials capable of employment in clandestine operations to control human behavior."[222] Congressional investigations have revealed how the scope of project MKULTRA widened from the use of drugs to many other techniques of controlling human behavior.

To mask the CIA's involvement in this research, the funding and organization of this program were carried out through tax-exempt foundations. As summarized in one Congressional investigation:

> The annual grants of funds to these specialists were made under ostensible research foundation auspices, thereby concealing the CIA's interest from the specialist's institution.[223]

Since the initial thrust of the MKULTRA program—successfully and covertly managed through civilian agencies—consisted of conducting biological weapons research, it is not hard to see that this clever technique of funding and controlling research could have been used after the biowarfare effort was allegedly shut down. After all, the biowarfare aspects of the program never received even the limited exposure that the mind control aspects of the program did. Additionally, the U.S. government successfully operated a covert radiation-testing program on its citizens in this manner. According to the *New York Times*, these experiments took place with the approval of the highest levels of government and were coordinated through a network of secret committees.[224] And these radiation experiments—which went on for decades—didn't come to light until the 1990s.

The same article mentioned above related the fact that in 1982 the U.S. Army was not only still actively involved with germ warfare and gene splicing research for "defensive" purposes (in spite of earlier bans) but also that it was sharing "vaccine" information with the World Health Organization. As related by the *Times*:

> The Army coordinates its research with the Centers for Disease Control in Atlanta and the World Health Organization, trying to come up with vaccines and treatment [sic] for the various infectious diseases.[225]

The fact that the WHO was working with the Fort Detrick cancer research/biowarfare facility should raise some concern in light of the allegations presented here concerning the role of the WHO in the international AIDS epidemic. Additional cause for concern is the revelation in this same article that the Fort Detrick researchers were also working with the Centers for Disease Control in Atlanta (the major U.S. clearinghouse for information on AIDS-related disease).

This close relationship between the CDC, WHO and the DOD was summed up by Joel Dalrymple of the virology division at Fort Detrick (in reference to the manner in which these organizations cooperated on vaccine development) as follows:

> The CDC, the World Health Organization (WHO), and DoD investigators have a long history of being able to work together in responding to requests for assistance from developing countries, to the benefit of all concerned.[226]

Dalrymple also stated:

> We keep the WHO informed. *I have many close colleagues working with the WHO, and there are many military persons working with the WHO or temporarily assigned to the WHO* since international health is one of our major concerns. We meet regularly with international scientists at scientific meetings, both informally and formally. *We openly provide information to all health agencies whenever there is an outbreak of disease,* such as a recent outbreak in Venezuela, and scientists from our laboratory have served as consultants and have worked very closely with the Pan-American Health

Organization, the WHO, and local scientists
investigating this outbreak. *We also maintain a
dialogue, and a collaborative interaction with
the Centers for Disease Control.*[227] [emphasis
added]

The close working relationship between WHO, the
CDC and the DOD "whenever there is an outbreak of
disease" internationally would provide the DOD with a
convenient means of controlling information in
response to an outbreak that might be the result of
biological warfare implemented by the DOD. By
supplying the right "experts" and consultants to WHO
and the CDC, the DOD could easily guide any
investigation into the cause of an *international*
epidemic and thereby obscure any role that the DOD
itself played in instigating an artificially created
epidemic. This level of control would be facilitated by
developments that have resulted not only in WHO
being put in charge of administering all international
programs related to the AIDS epidemic[228] but the U.S.
National Security Council declaring the HIV epidemic
to be a national security threat—thus giving the DOD
even more influence over the U.S. response to the
disease.[229]

Summary

A brief history has been presented of the following experimental themes in cancer vaccine research:

- The deliberate causation of cancer in human subjects through "cancer transplants" and the exploitation of immunosuppression by medical researchers in this research
- The development and use of immunosuppressive viruses resembling HIV for animal research designed specifically to increase cancer transplant growth and,
- The injection of human subjects of with cancer-causing animal viruses (including monkey cancer-causing viruses such as SV40) resulting in tumor formation.

The cooperation between cancer virus researchers, the WHO and the biowarfare communities has been noted, as has the recruitment of international war figures (with histories of mass human experimentation) by the U.S. biowarfare establishment. The profound utility of the AIDS epidemic to both the cancer virus research community and the biowarfare establishment has been documented.

These themes, along with the outbreak of the AIDS epidemic in humans shortly after similar diseases were induced in monkeys, and shortly after the causative agents were propagated in human cell cultures, prompt the following questions:

- Did the national security infrastructure working with cancer virus researchers and international war criminals cooperate to unleash deadly viruses developed in the war on cancer as a means of meeting national security-related depopulation goals?

- Has the world been turned into a giant concentration camp/pharmaceutical lab by war figures, with the inevitable deaths of its human population used to justify experimentation for the development of lucrative cancer vaccines?

For answers to be obtained to these and other questions posed in this study, an independent Congressional investigation would certainly be warranted. This inquiry should include an extensive investigation of the following: the history of human experimentation with cancer and immunosuppressive viruses by the cancer research community; the World Health Organization's hepatitis B cancer vaccine program; WHO's international smallpox vaccination program; the U.S. recruitment of Nazi and Japanese war figures and the post-war work they set about doing; and the national security goals for depopulating the Third World.

Such an investigation into the true cause of AIDS may set the record straight on how this deadly disease came to afflict the world population, and more specifically may be all that stands between unprecedented genocide and the Third World.

About the Author

Jerry Leonard is a physicist who has been actively involved in microelectronics research and production for over 15 years. He has been studying the documented history of cancer research, the development of immunosuppressive viruses and unethical government experimentation on human subjects—including the use of monkey cancer viruses—for over ten years.

[1] Luc Montagnier quoted in an interview in *Omni* magazine 12/88, pp. 102-134.

[2] V. Beral, H. Jaffe and R. Weiss, "Cancer Surveys: Cancer, HIV and AIDS," *Eur. J. Cancer*, vol. 27, no. 8, 1991, p. 1057.

[3] "Life expectancy in Africa cut short by AIDS," *CNN*; March 18, 1999; Web posted at: 12:24 p.m. EST (1724 GMT), WASHINGTON (CNN).

[4] Paul Ehrlich, *The Population Bomb*, (New York: Ballantine Books, 1968), p. 69.

[5] "Words of Clinton: 'Three Resolutions for the New Millennium,'" *New York Times*, 9/21/1999.

[6] These experiments were the continuation of a set of "cancer vaccine" experiments from the 1950s in which scientists inoculated human subjects with "tumor transplants" derived from processed cancer cells taken from other cancer patients. Such experiments resulted in tumors being induced in both healthy and sick human subjects. This line of experimentation was in turn the continuation of a similar line of research involving the creation of transplantable animal tumors and cancer viruses—all in the name of human cancer vaccine research.

[7] In the year 2000, 90% of AIDS deaths occurred in the Third World, the location where an alarmed National Security Council predicted in a classified 1974 pre-AIDS-era study that ninety percent of world population increases would occur by the year 2000, unless drastic measures were taken. As summarized in the declassified study: "Under the U.N. medium projection variant, by the year 2000 the population of less developed countries would double, rising from 2.5 billion to 5.0 billion. Thus, by the year 2000 ... over 90 percent of the annual increment to world population would occur there." *National Security Study Memorandum 200*, "Implications Of Worldwide Population Growth For U.S. Security And Overseas Interests," December 10, 1974 [Declassified 7/3/89], p. 17.

[8] As one researcher summarized, AIDS-related cancers are providing valuable insight into the cause of cancer in general: "The etiology and mechanism of the specific cancers that are

increased with HIV infection are proving highly informative for our general understanding of cancer etiology." C. Rabkin, "Epidemiology of AIDS-Related Malignancies," *Current Opinion in Oncology*, vol. 6, 1994, pp. 492-496.

[9] One influential writer referred to overpopulation as "the cancer of population growth" that "must be cut out." (Erlich) Militant environmentalists have referred to HIV as Mother Earth's immune system against people. Paul Erlich, *The Population Bomb*, (New York: Ballantine Books, 1968), Prologue.

[10] Lawrence K. Altman, "The Doctor's World: AIDS Research Yields Clues Linking Viruses and Cancer," *New York Times*, 4/14/98.

[11] It was this rapid increase in previously rare cancers—curiously those forms which were thought to have viral origins—which initially alerted doctors to the impending AIDS epidemic. As Lawrence Altman wrote in the *New York Times*: "It was the sudden appearance of the Kaposi's sarcoma cancer in large numbers of gay men in New York City that led doctors to recognize what is now called AIDS. Until then, Kaposi's sarcoma had been rare, and few experts suspected that it was related to a virus." Lawrence K. Altman, "Surviving With AIDS Is One Problem, Cancer Is Yet Another," *New York Times*, 5/6/97.

[12] In 1998, Denner made the following thought-provoking observation: "Although immunosuppression by retroviruses had already been described nearly 40 years ago, and although enormous efforts have been undertaken to study its mechanism because of the AIDS epidemic, the answer to how it works is still not known." J. Denner, "Immunosuppression by Retroviruses: Implications for Xenotransplantation," *Ann N Y Acad Sci.*, vol. 862, 1998 Dec. 30; pp. 75-86.

[13] One of these viruses, called the Duplan virus, was created by cancer researchers in 1962 by irradiating mouse leukemia viruses. According to an article published in 1989, this virus induces "a severe immunodeficiency disease with striking similarities to human AIDS." (Aziz) Other researchers who tested the nearly 40 year old virus reported: "This crude virus stock induced a severe immunodeficiency syndrome which has been designated murine

acquired immunodeficiency syndrome." (Huang) D. C. Aziz, Z. Hanna, P. Jolicoeur, "Severe Immunodeficiency Disease Induced by a Defective Murine Leukaemia Virus," *Nature*, vol. 338, 6 April 1988, pp. 505-508; M. Huang, P. Jolicoeur, "Characterization of the gag/Fusion Protein Encoded by the Defective Duplan Retrovirus Inducing Murine Acquired Immunodeficiency Syndrome," Journal of Virology, Dec. 1990, pp. 5764-5772.

[14] Through the sophisticated use of these viruses, cancer susceptibility could be increased by selectively destroying components of the immune system. Like the AIDS virus, some of these viruses were capable of selectively destroying a class of immune system cells, known as T-cells, in mice. See, for example: R. F. Mortensen, W. S. Ceglowski, H. Friedman, "Leukemia Virus-Induced Immunosuppression: Depression of T Cell-Mediated Cytotoxicity after Infection of Mice with Friend Leukemia Virus," *Journal of Immunology*, vol. 112, no. 6, June 1974, pp. 2077-2086.

[15] Researchers have estimated that more than 30% of AIDS victims develop cancer. Lawrence K. Altman, "Surviving With AIDS Is One Problem, Cancer Is Yet Another," *New York Times*, 5/6/97.

[16] Cancer researchers have long coveted the ability to watch cancer grow from its earliest stages in a large number of human subjects. To this end, human victims of naturally occurring immunosuppressive disorders have been the subject of numerous monitoring programs in which the relationship between immune system health and cancer could be correlated. (Good) By watching people predisposed to cancer, researchers could eliminate the drawbacks of epidemiological studies, in which such correlations were typically made after cancer had already been manifested. R. A. Good, "Relations Between Immunity and Malignancy," *Proc. Nat. Acad. Sci USA*, vol. 69, no. 4, April 1972, pp. 1026-1032.

[17] Vaccines to animal cancer viruses have been commercially available for some time.

[18] In 1980, researchers published a paper describing the "immunosuppressive activities" of several viruses when they were grown in cultures of human T-cells. One of these viruses was a baboon virus (BaEV) and one was a virus (called PMFV) derived from human cancers. J. Denner, V. Wunderlich, D. Bierwolf, "Suppression of human lymphocyte mitogen response by disrupted primate retroviruses of type C (baboon endogenous virus) and type D (PMFV)," *Acta Biol. Med. Germ.*, Band 39, K19-K26 (1980).

[19] A. Koike, G. E. Moore, C. B. Mendoza, A. L. Watne, "Heterologous, Homologous, and Autologous Transplantation of Human Tumors," *Cancer*, August, vol. 16, no. 8, 1963, pp. 1065-1071.

[20] These *human* experiments were modeled after *animal* experiments with these viruses. In one study, a monkey tumor virus was injected in a series of animal test subjects and then human test subjects used in a similar manner. *The monkey tumor virus was injected in human subjects and, after it induced "lesions" in the humans, subsequently recovered and passaged in other humans.* The researchers summarized their work, reminiscent of Nazi concentration camp studies in which viruses were passaged in humans used as living tissue cultures, as follows: "Finally, brief mention should be made of another interesting laboratory model. Feltz and Ambrus injected the virus into a number of common nonprimate laboratory animals, mice, rats, hamsters, rabbits, dogs, and cats, and found that none were susceptible. However, in subsequent studies, in conjunction with Ambrus and Feltz, we found that humans were susceptible, and responded with a proliferative lesion quite similar to that seen in the monkey. ... The human lesions were quite similar histologically to those of the monkey, however, the proliferative responses were less marked and regression of the nodules occurred within three to four weeks. The virus was readily recovered from the human lesions and serial passage, combined with viral titrations, demonstrated replication of the agent in the human." J. T. Grace, E. A. Mirand, S. J. Millian, R.S. Metzgar,

"Experimental Studies of Human Tumors," *Federation Proceedings*, January-February 1962, pp. 32-36.

[21] Researchers sought the mechanisms by which such viruses could inhibit human immune system functioning and how such viruses might cause human cancer. After determining that both monkey and human viruses had an "immunosuppressive effect" on T-cell function in human cell cultures, one group of researchers noted: "The possibility exists that immunosuppression induced by retroviruses in animal and man plays an important role in tumor progression and/or in establishing a generalized immunosuppressive state that predisposes the host to various infections." They also noted that "the mechanism and biological role of retroviral immunosuppression remain to be elucidated." Within a few years, the HIV would be supplying mountains of evidence that retroviruses can indeed play an important role in tumor progression in man. Robert Gallo would write in 1999 that "perhaps the most efficient virus in terms of fostering a high incidence of tumor development per infection is... of course, HIV-1." J. Denner, V. Wunderlich, D. Bierwolf, "Suppression of human lymphocyte mitogen response by disrupted primate retroviruses of type C (baboon endogenous virus) and type D (PMFV), *Acta Biol. Med. Germ.*, Band 39, K19-K26 (1980). R. Gallo, "Thematic Review Series XI: Viruses in the Origin of Human Cancer: Introduction and Overview," *Proceedings of the Association of American Physicians*, Vol. 111, Number 6, pp. 560-562.

[22] MPMV is one of "three independent virus isolates" of "simian acquired immunodeficiency syndrome (SAIDS) in macaque monkeys." As one group of researchers summarized: "When inoculated into young monkeys, MPMV produced a spectrum of nononcogenic disease associated with an immunodeficiency condition." Thayer RM, Power MD, Bryant ML, Gardner MB, Barr PJ, Luciw PA, "Sequence relationships of type D retroviruses which cause simian acquired immunodeficiency syndrome," *Virology*. 1987 Apr; 157(2), pp. 317-29.

[23] This immunosuppressive virus was isolated from a mammary tumor of a rhesus monkey in 1970. H. C. Chopra, M. M. Mason,

"A New Virus in a Spontaneous Mammary Tumor of a Rhesus Monkey," *Cancer Research*, vol. 30, No. 8, Aug. 1970, pp. 2081-2086.

[24] The virus not only had immunosuppressive properties, it was reported to act like a slow virus—just like HIV. D. L. Fine, J. Landon, R. Pienta, M. Kubicek, M. Valerio, W. Loeb, H. Chopra, "Responses of Infant Rhesus Monkeys to Inoculation With Mason-Pfizer Monkey Virus Materials," *Journal of the National Cancer Institute*, vol. 54 no. 3, March 1975, pp. 651-658.

[25] In 1986, one group of researchers described how immunodeficiency states were induced in monkeys in the early 1970s using MPMV. Since the virus did not immediately induce cancer, and since AIDS hadn't started in human populations, the effects of the virus (immunosuppression and fatal infection by opportunistic diseases), at that time, did not attract widespread notice. As the researchers summarized in one paper: "However the results were disappointing at that time because tumors were not induced by inoculation of MPMV into newborn rhesus monkeys and other nonhuman primates. Instead, many of the inoculated neonatal animals developed persistent lymphadenopathy, thymic atrophy, and weight loss and eventually died of undue susceptibility to facultative organisms. Because of the absence of transmissible tumor and the lack of occurrence at that time of human AIDS, this nononcogenic but immunosuppressive result attracted little scientific attention." M. L. Bryant, M. B. Gardner, P. A. Marx, D. H. Maul, N.W. Lerche, K. G. Osborn, L. J. Lowenstine, A. Bodgen, L. O. Arthur, E. Hunter, "Immunodeficiency in rhesus monkeys associated with the original Mason-Pfizer monkey virus," *J. Natl. Cancer Inst.*, 77(4), Oct 1986, pp. 957-65.

[26] Cryogenically preserved samples of this virus, isolated in the 1970s, were shown to induce a disease (simian acquired immune deficiency syndrome: SAIDS) very much like that due to simian immunodeficiency viruses (SIVs). As the researchers who published the experiment in 1986 summarized: "MPMV produces an acquired immunodeficiency similar to that caused by the recently described simian acquired immune deficiency syndrome

type D retroviruses." M. L. Bryant, M. B. Gardner, P. A. Marx, D. H. Maul, N.W. Lerche, K. G. Osborn, L. J. Lowenstine, A. Bodgen, L. O. Arthur, E. Hunter, "Immunodeficiency in rhesus monkeys associated with the original Mason-Pfizer monkey virus," *J. Natl. Cancer Inst.*, 77(4), Oct 1986, pp. 957-65.

[27] H. Ogura, T. Tanaka, M. Ocho, T. Kuwata, T. Oda, "Detection of Mason-Pfizer monkey virus infection by syncytia formation of human cells doubly transformed by Rous sarcoma virus and simian virus 40," *Arch Virol*, 57(2), 1978; pp. 195-8.

[28] Statement describing the massive scope of the CIA's previously secret program for testing drugs and other agents on the public under Project MKULTRA. See: "Project MKULTRA, The CIA's Program of Research In Behavioral Modification," *Joint Hearing Before the Select Committee on Intelligence and the Subcommittee on Health and Scientific Research of the Committee on Human Resources*, Ninety-Fifth Congress, First Session, August 3, 1977, p. 391.

[29] *Final Report of the Advisory Committee on Human Radiation Experiments*, October 21, 1994.

[30] With respect to the magnitude of this unethical experimentation, *The New York Times* recently revealed the following on its front page: "The President's committee found more than 4,000 experiments were conducted on as many as 20,000 individuals." Philip J. Hilts, "Secret Radioactive Experiments To Bring Compensation by U.S.," *New York Times*, 11/20/96.

[31] K. Schneider, "'50 Memo Shows Radiation Test Doubtful," *New York Times*, 12/28/94.

[32] Ibid.

[33] P. Hilts, "Panel Finds Wide Debate in 40's On the Ethics of Radiation Tests," *New York Times*, 10/12/94.

[34] Associated Press, "U.S. Released Atomic Cloud From a Rocket," *New York Times*, 8/25/94.

[35] Interim Report of the Advisory Committee on Human Radiation Experiments, October 21, 1994.

[36] S. Budiansky, E. E. Goode, T. Gest, "The Cold War Experiments," *U.S. News & World Report*, January 24, 1994, p.

34; "Project MKULTRA, The CIA's Program of Research In Behavioral Modification," p. 389.

[37] Among the Nazi chemist consultants employed by the Army Chemical Corps to supervise experiments on U.S. servicemen was one Otto Ambros, who was brought to the United States (where he was a consultant for W. R. Grace and Dow Chemical in addition to the government) even though he had been convicted as a war criminal (he was pardoned by John J. McCloy in 1951). Ambros was not only a director of the huge German chemical cartel I.G. Farben (which created the slave labor camp at Auschwitz) but "took part in the decision to use Zyklon B in the gas chambers." Linda Hunt, *Secret Agenda: The United States Government, Nazi Scientists, and Project Paperclip, 1945-1990*, (New York: St. Martin's Press, 1991), pp. 131-133.

[38] Warren E. Leary, "Experimental Drugs Linked To Ills of Gulf War Veterans," *New York Times*, 5/7/94.

[39] As Sheryl Gay Stolberg summarized in a *New York Times* article on the subject: "The Defense Department, acting with the food and drug agency's permission, gave the drug to more than 400,000 troops without obtaining their consent or telling them about potential risks." Sheryl Gay Stolberg, "Congressman Assails F.D.A. Decision on Drug for Gulf Troops," *New York Times*, 5/9/97.

[40] As Senator Rockefeller summarized during the opening of his congressional investigation: "During the Persian Gulf War, hundreds of thousands of soldiers were given experimental vaccines and drugs, and today we will hear evidence that these medical products could be causing many of the 'mysterious illnesses' those veterans are now experiencing." Opening Statement, Senator John D. Rockefeller IV, Chair Committee on Veterans' Affairs United States Senate; Hearing, "Is Military Research Hazardous to Veterans' Health? Lessons from the Cold War, the Persian Gulf, and Today," May 6, 1994.

[41] As the *New York Times* reported: "In 1990, the Defense Department got special waivers from the Food and Drug Administration to give drugs experimentally to U.S. troops. While some of the drugs were largely untested, others had been used

extensively, but for different purposes." Warren E. Leary, "Experimental Drugs Linked To Ills of Gulf War Veterans," *New York Times*, 5/7/94.

[42] Sheryl Gay Stolberg, "Congressman Assails F.D.A. Decision on Drug for Gulf Troops," *New York Times*, 5/9/97.

[43] R.W. Haley, T.L. Kurt, "Self-Reported Exposure to Neurotoxic Chemical Combinations in the Gulf War," JAMA, vol. 277, no. 3, January 15, 1997, pp. 231-237.

[44] As Warren Leary reported in the *New York Times*: "Senator John D. Rockefeller 4th, chairman of the Senate Veterans' Affairs Committee, said his committee's staff had spent six months looking into possible causes of the ailments reported by the veterans and had found a link with drugs experimentally given to more than 400,000 of the 700,000 troops who served in the war." Warren E. Leary, "Experimental Drugs Linked To Ills of Gulf War Veterans," *New York Times*, 5/7/94.

[45] *Preliminary Staff Findings* report (Committee on Veterans' Affairs United States Senate) sent to Senator Rockefeller by Diana Zuckerman and Patricia Olson, titled "Is Military Research Hazardous to Veterans' Health? Lessons from the Persian Gulf," May 6, 1994, pp. 5, 9.

[46] *Ibid.*, p. 8.

[47] *Ibid.*, p. 7.

[48] As a West Virginia (Rockefeller's home state) newspaper summarized in March of 1998: "Even though intelligence uncovered evidence that the Iraqis were prepared to use Sarin, rather than the other two agents, the Pentagon administered PB to all U.S. troops in the Gulf." This same paper quoted Senator Jay Rockefeller as saying: "The DOD has finally acknowledged that our troops were given a drug to protect against a nerve agent the enemy did not have. That this happened to our troops is very disturbing, That it took the DOD seven years to admit their error is inconceivable." Senator Rockefeller also stated that, "While it gravely disturbs me that the Pentagon recklessly exposed our troops to a potentially harmful mixture of chemicals during the Gulf War, I hold out some hope that they may have learned from

their errors." Mannix Porterfield, *The Register-Herald*, March 19, 1998.

[49] Is Military Research Hazardous to Veterans' Health?; Lessons Spanning Half a Century, A Staff Report Prepared for the Committee on Veterans' Affairs; United States Senate, December 8, 1994, 103d Congress, 2d Session, Committee Print - S. Prt. 103-97; JOHN D. ROCKEFELLER IV, West Virginia, Chairman, section: D. DOD USED INVESTIGATIONAL DRUGS IN THE PERSIAN GULF WAR IN WAYS THAT WERE NOT EFFECTIVE.

[50] As Philip Shenon related: "The files of the Defense Department and other Government agencies held extensive evidence suggesting that American soldiers had been exposed to Iraqi chemical weapons in the war, even as the Government assured the veterans and the public that no such evidence existed." Shenon continued: "After years of denials, the Pentagon now acknowledges that more than 20,000 troops may have been exposed when a battalion of American combat engineers blew up the Kamisiyah ammunition depot in the southern Iraqi desert in March 1991." A later study would reveal that this number was more likely closer to 100,000 troops. See: Philip Shenon, "Gulf War Ills Still Mystery Even After U.S. Shift on Gas Exposure," *New York Times*, 1/2/97; Philip Shenon, "House Committee Assails Pentagon On Gulf War Ills," *New York Times*, 10/26/97.

[51] Additionally, future CIA director John Deutch, while a top DOD official, appointed a Nobel Prize-winning scientist named Joshua Lederberg to the position of chairman of the Pentagon study group which ignored evidence of the exposure of US troops to chemical and biological warfare agents in the Gulf. Coincidentally, while serving in this position, Lederberg was simultaneously a director of an organization which had previously "made 70 Government-approved shipments of anthrax and other pathogens to Iraqi scientists." As summarized in an Associated Press report: "A scientist who headed a Pentagon study that dismissed exposure to chemical and biological agents as a cause of illness among Persian Gulf war veterans was a director of an organization that sent samples of deadly germs to Iraq before the

war began in January 1991, Newsday reported yesterday." Associated Press, "Report Ties Expert to Supplier of Germs to Iraq," *New York Times*, 11/28/96.

[52] Don Finley, 'Stealth' Germ Theory Invading Gulf War Illness Debate," *San Antonio Express-News*, 6/7/98.

[53] Don Finley, 'Stealth' Germ Theory Invading Gulf War Illness Debate," *San Antonio Express-News*, 6/7/98.

[54] Jesse Green, "Who Put the Lid On gp120?," *New York Times Magazine*, 3/26/95.

[55] Paul M. Rodriguez, "Sickness and Secrecy," *Insight Magazine*, Vol. 13, No. 31, Aug. 25, 1997; Paul M. Rodriguez, "The Gulf War Mystery," Vol. 13, No. 33, Sept. 8, 1997; Paul M. Rodriguez, "Gulf War Mystery and HIV," Vol. 13, No. 40, Nov. 3, 1997; Paul M. Rodriguez, "Breakthrough on Gulf War Illness," Vol. 15, No. 14, April 19, 1999.

[56] *Insight* quoted one of its sources for the story as follows: "First the DOD said they didn't have [squalene]; then they said they did but never used it; then they said they used it but only after the war; then they admitted they had manufactured it prior to the war but claimed they never used it; then it was confirmed that it has been used overseas in trials for a number of years; then, well, you get the picture."

[57] It is possible that researchers used the potential offensive use of HIV-related biowarfare agents by the Iraqis as an excuse for testing alleged experimental HIV vaccines on US troops. The attempt to convert HIV to a biological warfare agent by a foreign government is not without precedent. A top-level Soviet defector has claimed in a recent book that the Soviets experimented with the use of HIV as a biowarfare agent. See: William J. Broad and Judith Miller, "Defector Tells of Soviet and Chinese Germ Weapons," *New York Times*, 4/5/99.

[58] Paul Brown, "Illegal vaccine link to Gulf war syndrome," *Guardian*, 7/30/01.

[59] This research, which was similar to that conducted in the concentration camps in Nazi Germany, included experiments in which soldiers were given experimental protective measures against a pathogen and then deliberately exposed to the pathogen,

so that the efficacy of the experimental treatment could be directly evaluated. Consider the following account of early biowarfare research conducted at Fort Detrick: "Human experimentation using military and civilian volunteers was initiated in 1955. Biological munitions were detonated inside a 1-million-liter, hollow, metallic, spherical aerosolization chamber at Fort Detrick known as the 'eight ball.' Volunteers inside the chamber were exposed to Francisella tularensis and Coxiella burnetii. These and other challenge studies were done to determine vulnerability to aerosolized pathogens and the efficacy of vaccines, prophylaxis, and therapies under development." See G. W. Christopher, T. J. Cieslak, J. A. Pavlin, E. M. Eitzen, "Biological Warfare: A Historical Perspective," *JAMA*, August 6, 1997, Vol. 278, No. 5, pp. 412-417.

[60] R. J. Benjamin, H. Waldmann, "Induction of Tolerance by Monoclonal Antibody Therapy," *Nature*, vol. 320, April 3, 1986, p. 449.

[61] The similarities between these viruses and HIV include the selective targeting and destruction of T-cells. For an early (pre-AIDS) study published on the creation and testing of a mouse immunosuppressive virus which selectively destroys the immune systems of mice in a manner suspiciously similar to human HIV, see: M. Lieberman, S. Segal, O. Finn, I. Zan-Bar, S. Kaplan, "Differential Effects of Radiation Leukemia Virus Infection on the Immunobiology of C57BL/Ka Mice," in Ed. J. F. Duplan, *Radiation-Induced Leukemogenesis and Related Viruses*, (Elsevier/North-Holland Publishing Company, 1977), pp. 115-125.

[62] Contrary to public perception, immunosuppressive viruses have been used for decades in the cancer research community to systematically increase susceptibility to cancer for experimental purposes. The devastating characteristics of infection with these viruses have also been understood by a narrow group of scientists for some time. One researcher summarizing the ongoing research into the occurrence of the feline acquired immunodeficiency syndrome (or FAIDS) in cats noted that "the whole immunodeficiency picture became well recognised long before

AIDS was found in humans." W. F. H. Jarrett, "Cancer and AIDS; the Contribution of Comparative Medicine," *The Veterinary Record*, July 2, 1988, p. 35.

[63] For an early experiment of this type, see: M. A. Chirigos, K. Perk, W. Turner, B. Burka, M. Gomez, "Increased Oncogenicity of the Murine Sarcoma Virus (Moloney) by Co-infection with Murine Leukemia Viruses," *Cancer Research*, vol. 28, June 1968, pp. 1055-1063.

[64] A. Peled, N. Haran-Ghera, "Immunosuppression by the Radiation Leukemia Virus and its Relation to Lymphatic Leukemia Development," *Int. J. Cancer*, vol. 8, pp. 97-106.

[65] Mouse AIDS is often referred to as MAIDS.

[66] These goals were eventually met in animal cancer research due, in part, to the experimental use of immunosuppressive viruses. According to some researchers, these goals may soon be met in human cancer research thanks to the Human Immunodeficiency Virus epidemic. See section entitled "The Benefits of the AIDS Epidemic" in this report.

[67] These cancer viruses were derived from experiments in which scientists succeeded in inducing cancer in lab animals from filtered extracts of cancerous tissue. (These cancerous tissues were typically derived from cancers induced through exposure of other lab animals to chemicals and radiation.) See: Ludwik Gross, *Oncogenic Viruses* (Oxford: Pergamon Press, 1983), p. 321.

[68] Cancer researchers recently obtained this goal in animal research using the HIV virus! In this case HIV was used both to cause and prevent cancer growth in mice. By adapting HIV for growth in animal cells, model tumors were formed in mice. By using HIV in the creation of a vaccine, researchers could inhibit the growth of these tumors. By using mice with various immune system deficiencies, researchers were able to dissect the immune response to these cancer viruses. As the researchers summarized this experiment and its results: "Using a tumor expressing HIV gp160 as a model viral tumor... we found a growth-regression-recurrence pattern, and used this to investigate mechanisms of immunosurveillance. In this study, we present a novel manipulable animal model of tumor immunosurveillance in which

we can evaluate escape mechanisms of tumor cells from immunosurveillance, the role of CD8+ T cells in causing regression and preventing local recurrence and the adverse role of CD4+ T cells in local recurrence." S. Matsui, J. Ahlers, A. Vortmeyer, M. Terabe, T. Tsukui, D. Carbone, L. Liotta, J. Berzofsky, "A Model for CD8+ CTL Tumor Immunosurveillance and Regulation of Tumor Escape by CD4 T Cells Through an Effect on Quality of CTL," *Journal of Immunology*, vol. 163, no.1, July 1, 1999, pp. 184-193.

[69] See G. R. Minot, R. Isaacs, "Transfusion of Lymphocytes," *J.A.M.A.*, vol. 84, no. 23, pp. 713-15.

[70] See: H. B. Stone, "Danger of Implanting Tumor Cells in Human Beings for the Purpose of 'Immunization,'" Letters to the Editor, *Annals of Surgery*, vol. 135, no. 5, May, 1952, p. 753.

[71] The results of these tests were found to be encouraging for those hoping to use such immune modulating procedures as a method of treating or preventing cancer. See: C. M. Southam, A. Brunschwig, A. G. Levin, Q. S. Dizon, "Effect of Leukocytes on Transplantability of Human Cancer," *Cancer*, Nov. 1966, pp. 1743-1753; A. Brunschwig, C. M. Southam, A. G. Levin, "Host Resistance to Cancer," *Annals of Surgery*, vol. 162, no. 3, Sept. 1965, pp. 416-425.

[72] C. M. Southam, L. Pillemer, "Serum Properdin Levels and Cancer Cell Homografts in Man," *Proceedings Soc. of Experimental Biology and Medicine (P.S.E.B.M.)*, vol. 96, pp. 596-601.

[73] C. M. Southam, A. E. Moore, "Clinical Studies of Viruses as Antineoplastic Agents, With Particular Reference to Egypt 101 Virus," *Cancer*, vol. 5, 1952, p. 1033.

[74] It is somewhat ironic that Southam's work with anti-cancer viruses caused him to wish for immunosuppressive agents that would eventually be used to allow cancer to grow more effectively.

[75] Alternatively natural sources of immunosuppression capable of aiding cancer growth could be eliminated. This would provide a natural form of cancer prevention by allowing the body's own unimpaired immunologic processes to reject cancer growth.

[76] Researchers used cancer viruses for the animal cancer transplant experiments because such viruses had been discovered through experiments with cancer cell transplants. In contrast, the human studies with cancer transplants used processed *cells* from human tumors because no definitive human cancer viruses had yet been identified in these cells.

[77] S. Kaufmann, C. Ladel, "Application of knockout mice to the experimental analysis of infections with bacteria and protozoa." *Trends in Microbiology*, vol. 2, no. 7, July 1994, pp. 235-42.

[78] As one group of researchers recently summarized: "Improvement of T Cell-mediated immunity for immunotherapy and development of vaccines has been one of the major strategies against cancer in this decade." S. Matsui, J. Ahlers, A. Vortmeyer, M. Terabe, T. Tsukui, D. Carbone, L. Liotta, J. Berzofsky, "A Model for CD8+ CTL Tumor Immunosurveillance and Regulation of Tumor Escape by CD4 T Cells Through an Effect on Quality of CTL," *Journal of Immunology*, vol. 163, no.1, July 1, 1999, pp. 184-193.

[79] M. Woodruff, N. Dunbar, A. Ghaffar, "The growth of tumours in T-cell deprived mice and their response to treatment with Corynebacterium parvum," *Proc. R. Soc. Lond. B*, vol. 184, pp. 97-102 (1973).

[80] Researchers studied the response to cancer cell implants in healthy animals (controls), immunosuppressed animals and immunosuppressed animals that also received "vaccines" consisting of irradiated cancer cell injections and bacteria.

[81] Since the immunosuppressive treatment itself *reduced* the growth of cancer relative to healthy controls in these studies, scientists suspected that by destroying subpopulations of T-cells (helper T-cells) through immunosuppression, the immune system was indirectly *stimulated* to fight the cancer. (Destroying certain classes of T-cells may have reduced their ability to cause other immune system cells to spread cancer growth. This result was found in numerous other experiments of this type.) Alternatively, the even more positive effect of the vaccine in combination with the immunosuppressive treatments could have been due to other immune system cells, such as stimulated macrophages. As the

researchers summarized: "This appears to lend support to the hypothesis that the antitumour effect of C. parvum depends primarily on macrophage stimulation." M. Woodruff, N. Dunbar, A. Ghaffar, "The growth of tumours in T-cell deprived mice and their response to treatment with Corynebacterium parvum," *Proc. R. Soc. Lond. B*, vol. 184, pp. 97-102.

[82] W. S. Ceglowski, H. Friedman, "Immunosuppression by Leukemia Viruses," *Journal of Immunology*, vol. 101, no. 3, 1968, pp. 594-604.

[83] L. J. Anderson, W.F. H. Jarrett, O. Jarrett, H. M. Laird, "Feline Leukemia-Virus Infection of Kittens: Mortality Associated With Atrophy of the Thymus and Lymphoid Depletion," *J. Nat. Cancer Inst.*, vol. 47, 1971, pp. 807-817; L. E. Perryman, E. A. Hoover, D. S. Yohn, "Immunologic Reactivity of the Cat: Immunosuppression in Experimental Feline Leukemia," *J. Natl. Cancer Inst.*, vol. 49, 1972, pp. 1357-1365.

[84] All of these methods were used in conjunction with transplants of cancer to determine how a defective immune system aided cancer growth relative to healthy animal subjects.

[85] For a description of an experiment of this type in mice, see: M. A. Chirigos, K. Perk, W. Turner, B. Burka, M. Gomez, "Increased Oncogenicity of the Murine Sarcoma Virus (Moloney) by Co-infection with Murine Leukemia Viruses," *Cancer Research*, vol. 28, June 1968, pp. 1055-1063.

[86] Using methods similar to those used in experiments which were conducted with *mice* using combinations of leukemia and other cancer viruses, experiments were also conducted with *cats* from the early 1970s in which attenuated or inactivated feline leukemia viruses were used to induce immunosuppression in combination with cancer virus injections. Following the induction of immunosuppression with the modified feline leukemia virus, experimental cats were found to be much more susceptible to cat cancer viruses. See: R. G. Olsen, E. A. Hoover, J. P. Schaller, L. E. Mathes, L. H. Wolff, "Abrogation of Resistance to Feline Oncornavirus Disease by Immunization with Killed Feline Leukemia Virus," *Cancer Research*, vol. 37, July 1977, pp. 2082-2085.

[87] This research had an added benefit over the immunosuppressive research with chemicals, surgery and radiation treatments. It allowed scientists to test a more realistic theory of how viral cancer occurred in nature. Since it was suspected that naturally occurring immunosuppressive viruses aided cancer growth due to cancer viruses, researchers could test the validity of this hypothesis by injecting immunosuppressive viruses that they manufactured in combination with cancer injections.

[88] For example, decades of experimentation involving suppression of T-cells through immunosuppression showed that T-cells were instrumental in preventing cancer. Researchers are now making breakthroughs in "priming" the T-cell response to cancer in both animals and humans as a means of preventing cancer. See: C. J. M. Melief, W. M. Kast, "Lessons from T Cell Responses to Virus Induced Tumours for Cancer Eradication in General," *Cancer Surveys*, vol. 13, pp. 81-99.

[89] For an overview of the immunosuppressive viruses used in this type of research and their various effects on the immune system, see: P. B. Dent, "Immunodepression by Oncogenic Viruses," *Progr. med. Virol.*, vol. 14, 1972, pp. 1-35.

[90] For an overview of the progress made in animal cancer vaccines over the last few decades, see: M. R. Hilleman, "Historical and Contemporary Perspectives in Vaccine Developments: From the Vantage of Cancer," *Prog Med Virol.*, vol. 39, pp. 1-18.

[91] For an overview of these cancer cell injection experiments, see: E. Langer, "Human Experimentation: Cancer Studies at Sloan-Kettering Stir Public Debate on Medical Ethics," *Science*, vol. 143, 7 February, 1964, pp. 551-553; C. M. Southam, "Homotransplantation of Human Cell Lines," *Bull. N.Y. Acad. Med.*, vol. 34, no. 6, June 1958, pp. 416-23.

[92] N. Tanigaki, C. M. Southam, "Use of an Indirect Antiglobulin Consumption Test to Detect Isoantibodies Following Human Cancer Cell Homotransplants," *Europ. J. Cancer,* vol. 2, pp. 143-156; T. Itoh, C. M. Southam, "Isoantibodies to Human Cancer Cells in Healthy Recipients of Cancer Homotransplants," *J. Immun.*, vol. 91, 1963, pp. 469-483; C. M. Southam, L. Pillemer, "Serum Properdin Levels and Cancer Cell Homografts in Man,"

Proceedings Soc. of Experimental Biology and Medicine (P.S.E.B.M.), vol. 96, pp. 596-601.

[93] A. E. Levin, D. B. Custodio, E. E. Mandel, C. M. Southam, "Rejection of Cancer Homotransplants by Patients With Debilitating Non-Neoplastic Diseases," *Annals New York Academy of Sciences,* vol. 120, 1964, pp. 410-423.

[94] At least 300 healthy humans were eventually exposed to cancer cell injections in this set of experiments. C. M. Southam, "The Immunological Status of Patients with Nonlymphomatous Cancer," *Cancer Research*, vol. 28, July 1968, p. 1437.

[95] Since cancer patients demonstrated a much greater susceptibility to induced tumors than healthy patients or patients with diseases other than cancer, the researchers assumed this was because the cancer patients had a specific immune system deficiency that had resulted in their contracting cancer. Southam described this phenomenon as follows: "The tumor inoculums survived for longer periods in patients with more advanced cancer. *These observations could be explained by variations in the immunological responses of the hosts.*" [emphasis added] C. M. Southam, "Homotransplantation of Human Cell Lines," *Bull. N.Y. Acad. Med.*, vol. 34, no. 6, June 1958, pp. 416-23.

[96] Healthy patients who were given repeat injections of cancer cells became less susceptible to tumors from these injections. This development was viewed as a primitive form of vaccine or acquired immunity to cancer. As Southam summarized:

"The growth of a repeat implant of the same cell type has been studied in normal recipients. The repeated implants formed smaller nodules and regressed more rapidly as judged by gross and microscopic examination. *This accelerated rejection of a second implant is presumably the result of an induced immunity.*" [emphasis added]

C. M. Southam, "Homotransplantation of Human Cell Lines," *Bull. N.Y. Acad. Med.*, vol. 34, no. 6, June 1958, pp. 416-23. See also: C. M. Southam, A. E. Moore, "Induced Immunity to Cancer

Cell Homografts in Man," *Annals of New York Academy of Sciences*, vol. 73, 1958, p. 635.

[97] A. Koike, G. E. Moore, C. B. Mendoza, A. L. Watne, "Heterologous, Homologous, and Autologous Transplantation of Human Tumors," *Cancer*, August, vol. 16, no. 8, 1963, pp. 1065-1071.

[98] L. Gross, "Is Leukemia Caused by a Transmissable Virus?," *Blood: The Journal of Hematology*, vol. IX, No. 6, June, 1954, p. 565.

[99] Cobbold, Jayasuriya, Nash, Prospero, Waldmann, "Therapy with Monoclonal Antibodies by Elimination of T-cell Subsets *in vivo*," *Nature*, vol. 312, 1984, pp. 548-551; H. Friedman, W. S. Ceglowski, "Cellular Basis for the Immunosuppressive Properties of a Leukaemogenic Virus," *Nature*, vol. 218, June 29, 1968, pp. 1232-1234.

[100] J. Gordon, "The B Lymphocyte-Deprived Mouse As a Tool in Immunobiology," *Journal of Immunological Methods*, vol. 25, 1979, pp. 227-238.

[101] As one group of researchers noted in an article published in the *Bulletin of the World Health Organization*: "Recent studies on virus-induced immunopathological reactions in domestic and experimental animals have led to the development of concepts and technical methods that may be useful in investigating certain viral diseases in man ..." A. Allison, W. Beveridge, W. Cockburn, J. East, H. Goodman, H. Koprowski, P. Lambert, J Van Loghem, P. Miescher, C. Mimms, A. Notkins, G. Torrigiani, "Virus-Associated Immunopathology: Animal Models and Implications For Human Disease," *Bulletin of the World Health Organization*, vol. 47, no. 2, 1972, p. 258.

[102] The link between the "contaminated" vaccine and the immunosuppressive effect would have to remain hidden. This could be accomplished by choosing a virus with a long incubation period so that a correlation between the vaccine and the resultant epidemic would not be readily made. If such a link was eventually made, the use of experimental immunosuppressive viruses that could appear to be "accidental" contaminants of the vaccine

would allow researchers to conduct such an experiment with impunity.

[103] Most likely the experiment would be conducted through the injection of animal immunosuppressive viruses adapted for human cell growth in human subjects to deliberately increase susceptibility to cancer in human subjects. The bovine immunosuppressive virus (BIV), which causes immunosuppression in cattle, was adapted for human cell growth in the 1970s before the outbreak of AIDS in human populations. (Georgiades) Bovine lentiviruses similar to BIV were initially correlated with one strain of HIV in human AIDS patients. (Shaw) In addition to bovine viruses, monkey immunosuppressive viruses were also modified for growth in human cells. The Baboon virus (BaEV) and the immunosuppressive monkey virus MPMV, were grown in human cell cultures, along with similar human viruses, to measure their immunosuppressive properties just before the AIDS epidemic exploded in human populations. J. A. Georgiades, A. Billiau, B. Vanderschueren, "Infection of Human Cell Cultures with Bovine Visna Virus," *J. gen. Virol.* (1978), 38, pp. 375-380; G. M. Shaw, M. E. Harper, B. H. Hahn, L. G. Epstein, D. C. Gajdusek, R. W. Price, B. A. Navia, C. K. Petito, C. J. O'Hara, J. E. Groopman, E. S. Cho, J. M. Oleske, F. Wong-Staal, R. C. Gallo, "Sequence Homology and Morphologic Similarity of HTLV-III and Visna Virus, a Pathogenic Lentivirus," *Science.* vol. 227, 11 January 1985, pp. 173-182.

[104] Such monitoring could be conducted under the humanitarian pretext of fighting AIDS-related illnesses. *This would effectively allow scientists to conduct cancer research under the pretext of providing clinical care for AIDS patients.* Similar large-scale monitoring efforts were undertaken to determine how radiation affected the human body during the Cold War when government scientists secretly monitored uranium miners and the population of the Marshall Islands who were deliberately exposed to radioactive materials during the course of government weapons programs. With respect to the uranium miners, a recent government report summarized: "The miners, who were the subject of government study as they mined uranium for use in

weapons manufacturing, were subject to radon exposures well in excess of levels known to be hazardous. The government failed to act to require the reduction of the hazard by ventilating the mines, and it failed to adequately warn the miners of the hazard to which they were being exposed, even though such actions would likely have posed no threat to the national security." With respect to the Marshallese, the same report noted: "The exposed Marshallese population received additional doses of radiation from later bomb tests and residual radiation in the food chain, which continues to this day. The U.S. government ... has provided care to the Marshallese ever since for radiation-related illnesses while conducting research on this population to determine radiation effects. *For many years the distinction between research and clinical care was not adequately explained to the Marshallese.*" [emphasis added] Chapter 17, *Final Report of the Advisory Committee on Human Radiation Experiments*, October 21, 1994.

[105] Such a procedure would allow researchers to "predispose" human subjects to cancer growth and then monitor cancer growth in its earliest phases, in a large number of people. The advantage of such an opportunity, over the drawbacks of other indirect, drawn-out epidemiological cancer studies, was noted by one researcher in the following manner: "Future attempts at identifying etiologic agents in human leukemia and lymphoma may involve the longitudinal study of individuals over a period of time that covers the critical phase of tumor induction. Such a project would be extremely difficult to carry out, perhaps impossible, if all persons had an identical risk of developing these otherwise uncommon cancers. Epidemiologic and experimental advantages would result from the use of patients at exceptionally high risk of leukemia and lymphoma, such as those affected with certain constitutional diseases." AIDS is providing just such an ideal disease state in humans which allows researchers to watch a group of "patients at exceptionally high risk of leukemia and lymphoma" before, during and after their immune systems conveniently self-destruct. J. P. Fraumeni, Jr., "Constitutional Disorders of Man Predisposing to Leukemia and Lymphoma,"

National Cancer Institute Monograph 32, August 1969, pp. 221-232.

[106] Homosexuals were likely chosen for this experiment because studies had shown that homosexual populations disproportionately harbored latent infections of numerous viruses that were assumed to be capable of causing cancer. This fact would allow researchers to conduct experiments similar to those conducted in animals by using only injections of immunosuppressive viruses. (This is discussed in a later section of this study.) It is also possible that controlled amounts of cancer viruses were included in this vaccine so that correlations could be made between the progress of cancer growth and the degree of immunosuppression and amount of cancer the subjects were exposed to. The use of such a procedure would merely be a more sophisticated form of the experiment described below in which immunosuppressed cancer patients were injected with tumor-causing animal cancer viruses such as SV40.

[107] W. Szmuness, C. E. Stevens, E. J. Harley, E. A. Zang, W. R. Oleszko, D. C. William, R. Sadovsky, J. M. Morrison, A. Kellner, "Hepatitis B Vaccine: Demonstration of Efficacy in a Controlled Clinical Trial in a High-Risk Population in the United States," *The New England Journal of Medicine*, vol. 303, no. 15, October 9, 1980, p. 834.

[108] G. J. P. Van Griensven, N. A. Hessol, B. A. Koblin, R. H. Byers, P. M. O'Malley, N. Albrecht-van Lent, S. P. Buchbinder, P. E. Taylor, C. E. Stevens, R. A. Coutinho, "Epidemiology of Human Immunodeficiency Virus Type 1 Infection among Homosexual Men Participating in Hepatitis B Vaccine Trials in Amsterdam, New York City, and San Francisco, 1978-1990," *American Journal of Epidemiology*, vol. 137, no. 8, p. 913.

[109] Studies show that 40% of the recipients of some of these vaccine trials developed AIDS. (Half of the volunteers participating in these trials were given a placebo.) See: C. E. Stevens, P. E. Taylor, E. A. Zang, J. M. Morrison, E. J. Harley, S. Rodriguez de Cordoba, C. Bacino, R. C. Y. Ting, A. J. Bodner, M. G. Sarngadharan, R. C. Gallo, P. Rubinstein, "Human T-Cell Lymphotropic Virus Type III Infection in a Cohort of

Homosexual Men in New York City," *JAMA*, April 25, 1986, vol. 255, no. 16, pp. 2167-2172; G. J. P. Van Griensven, N. A. Hessol, B. A. Koblin, R. H. Byers, P. M. O'Malley, N. Albrecht-van Lent, S. P. Buchbinder, P. E. Taylor, C. E. Stevens, R. A. Coutinho, "Epidemiology of Human Immunodeficiency Virus Type 1 Infection among Homosexual Men Participating in Hepatitis B Vaccine Trials in Amsterdam, New York City, and San Francisco, 1978-1990," *American Journal of Epidemiology*, vol. 137, no. 8, pp. 913.

[110] D. W. Lyter, J. Bryant, R. Thackeray, C. R. Rinaldo, L. A. Kingsley, "Incidence of Human Immunodeficiency Virus-Related and Nonrelated Malignancies in a Large Cohort of Homosexual Men," *J. Clin. Oncol.*, Oct. 1995, vol. 13, no. 10, pp. 2540-6; C. R. Rinaldo, L. A. Kingsley, D. W. Lyter, B. S. Rabin, R. W. Atchison, A. J. Bodner, S. H. Weiss, W. C. Saxinger, "Association of HTLV-III with Epstein Barr Virus Infection and Abnormalities of T Lymphocytes in Homosexual Men," *Journal of Infectious Diseases*, vol. 154, no. 4, October 1986, pp. 556-561.

[111] The hepatitis vaccine developed in these trials has been referred to by some observers as the first human cancer vaccine.

[112] As researchers affiliated with the WHO noted in one publication: "The Meeting considered that there were good grounds to suppose that vaccination of children with hepatitis B vaccine at birth, or shortly thereafter, would confer long-term protection against the development of hepatocellular carcinoma." "Prevention of Liver Cancer," *World Health Organization Technical Report Series 691*, (Geneva: World Health Organization, 1983), p. 27.

[113] These cancer vaccine trials have been declared a success. As one paper put it: "Universal childhood vaccination against hepatitis B in Taiwan appears to have reduced the incidence of hepatocellular carcinoma." Mei-Hwei Chang, Chien-Jen Chen, Mei- Shu Lai, Hsu-Mei Hsu, Tzee-Chung Wu, Man-Shan Kong, Der-Cherng Liang, Wen-Yi Shau, Ding-Shinn Chen "Universal hepatitis B vaccination in Taiwan and the incidence of hepatocellular carcinoma in children." *The New England Journal of Medicine*, June 26, 1997 vol. 336 no. 26, p. 1855.

[114] This process might allow long-term *immunocompetence* (through vaccine development) to be attained through short-term *immunocompromise* induced in a group of unfortunate human test subjects.

[115] This procedure would also represent the replication in human populations of an experiment conducted in cats in which kittens were injected with a "vaccine" containing a mixture of immunosuppressive viruses and cancer agents. As the authors of this study summarized: "Four-week-old specific-pathogen-free cats were immunized with a combined vaccine composed of killed feline leukemia virus and killed feline oncornavirus-associated cell membrane antigen-containing tumor cells." The authors of this study explained that the immunosuppressive leukemia virus present in the vaccine increased susceptibility to the cancer agents: "Thus, it appears that the protective immunity to feline oncornavirus disease was hindered rather than enhanced by inclusion of inactivated, purified FeLV as a vaccine component." R. G. Olsen, E. A. Hoover, J. P. Schaller, L. E. Mathes, L. H. Wolff, "Abrogation of Resistance to Feline Oncornavirus Disease by Immunization with Killed Feline Leukemia Virus," *Cancer Research*, vol. 37, July 1977, pp. 2082-2085.

[116] Pearce Wright, "Smallpox vaccine 'triggered Aids virus,'" *The Times of London*, Monday, May 11, 1987

[117] The following chilling recommendation for future research was made in a World Health Organization publication from 1972: *"An attempt should be made to ascertain whether viruses can in fact exert selective effects on immune function ... or by affecting T cell function as opposed to B cell function.* The possibility should also be looked into that the immune response to the virus may itself be impaired *if the infecting virus damages more or less selectively the cells responding to the viral antigens."* [emphasis added] This is exactly what HIV does. A. Allison, W. Beveridge, W. Cockburn, J. East, H. Goodman, H. Koprowski, P. Lambert, J Van Loghem, P. Miescher, C. Mimms, A. Notkins, G. Torrigiani, "Virus-Associated Immunopathology: Animal Models and Implications For Human Disease," *Bulletin of the World Health Organization*, vol. 47, no. 2, 1972, p. 259.

[118] "Recent studies on virus-induced immunopathological reactions in domestic and experimental animals have led to the development of concepts and technical methods that may be useful in investigating certain viral diseases in man, including hepatitis." [emphasis added] *Bulletin of the World Health Organization*, vol. 47, no. 2, 1972, p. 258.

[119] "In relation to the immune response, *a number of useful experimental approaches can be visualized. One would be a study of the relationship of HL-A type to the immune response, both humoral and cellular, to well-defined bacterial and viral antigens during preventive vaccination.*" [emphasis added] *Federation Proceedings*, vol. 31, no. 3, May-June, 1972, p. 1102.

[120] The pre-AIDS WHO report recommended that an "... international co-operative study of patients with *immunological deficiency syndromes* should be carried out." It also suggested that "[o]bservations on patients with immunological deficiency diseases should be as complete as possible, and it is desirable that they should enable valid comparisons to be made between patients studied in different institutions." [emphasis added] A. C. Allison, B. A. Askonas, B. Benacerraf, R. Ceppellini, R.A. Good, E. S. Lennox, H. O. McDevitt, R. S. Nezlin, M. Seligmann, "Genetics of the Immune Response," *World Health Organization Technical Report Series*, No. 402, pp. 34, 52.

[121] As one group of researchers summarized: "Thus the AIDS epidemic is providing a natural experiment on a massive scale from which much can be learned about the role of immunosuppression in the development of cancer." V. Beral, H. Jaffe and R. Weiss, "Cancer Surveys: Cancer, HIV and AIDS," *Eur. J. Cancer*, vol. 27, no. 8, 1991, p. 1057.

[122] This theory has been referred to as the "immune-surveillance" theory of cancer development. That is, when the immune system can no longer conduct surveillance to eliminate cancer cells, tumors can grow uncontrollably. Such a mechanism involving simultaneously exposure to immune system depressing malaria in conjunction with the Epstein-Barr virus was thought to be responsible for Burkitt's lymphoma in human populations.

Curiously Burkitt's lymphoma is one of the chief forms of cancer which develops in AIDS patients.

[123] In an ironic twist, the ballooning numbers of immunosuppressed AIDS victims which will provide this vital information may also serve both as test vehicles for experimental cancer vaccines as well as a huge and lucrative market for the eventual sale of such revolutionary vaccines.

[124] E. Langer, "Human Experimentation: Cancer Studies at Sloan-Kettering Stir Public Debate on Medical Ethics," *Science*, vol. 143, pp. 551-553.

[125] A. Koike, G. E. Moore, C. B. Mendoza, A. L. Watne, "Heterologous, Homologous, and Autologous Transplantation of Human Tumors," *Cancer*, August, vol. 16, no. 8, 1963, pp. 1065-1071.

[126] In describing the results of one of his experiments with cancer cell transplants, Southam noted that one group of recipients of these cancer injections "were receiving anticancer chemotherapy or radiotherapy which might have an additional immunosuppressive effect." C. M. Southam, A. Brunschwig, A. G. Levin, Q. S. Dizon, "Effect of Leukocytes on Transplantability of Human Cancer," *Cancer*, Nov. 1966, p. 1750.

[127] C. M. Southam, A. Brunschwig, A. G. Levin, Q. S. Dizon, "Effect of Leukocytes on Transplantability of Human Cancer," *Cancer*, Nov. 1966, p. 1753.

[128] By watching only those patients known to be predisposed to cancer growth due to naturally occurring immunodeficiencies, the observation time required could be drastically shortened in crucial experiments designed to monitor tumor growth from its very beginning stages. These advantages (for naturally occurring forms of immunodeficiencies) were summarized by Joseph Fraumeni in a National Cancer Institute Monograph (cited earlier) as follows:

"Future attempts at identifying etiologic agents in human leukemia and lymphoma may involve the longitudinal study of individuals over a period of time that covers the critical phase of tumor induction. Such a project would be extremely difficult to carry out, perhaps impossible, if all persons had an identical risk of developing these otherwise uncommon cancers. *Epidemiologic and experimental advantages would result from the use of patients at exceptionally high risk of leukemia and lymphoma, such as those affected with certain constitutional diseases.*" [emphasis added]

Fraumeni also noted, "There are significant advantages to the use of constitutional disorders and other 'high-risk' conditions in laboratory and epidemiologic research on these neoplasms." One of these advantages was that researchers could probe the immune responses of such patients and then correlate the exact form of their deficiencies with cancer growth. J. P. Fraumeni, Jr., "Constitutional Disorders of Man Predisposing to Leukemia and Lymphoma," *National Cancer Institute Monograph 32*, August 1969, p. 228.

[129] J. A. Georgiades, A. Billiau, B. Vanderschueren, "Infection of Human Cell Cultures with Bovine Visna Virus," *J. gen. Virol.* (1978), 38, pp. 375-380.

[130] P. Sonigo, C. Barker, E. Hunter, S. Wain-Hobson, "Nucleotide Sequence of Mason-Pfizer Monkey Virus: An Immuosuppressive D-Type Retrovirus," *Cell*, vol. 45, May 9, 1986, pp. 375-385.

[131] H. Ogura, M. Ocho, T. Tanaka, T. Oda, "Susceptibility of Human Cultured Cells to Mason-Pfizer Monkey Virus," *Gann*, vol. 69, June, 1978, pp. 413-415; H. Ogura, T. Tanaka, M. Ocho, M. Namba, T. Oda, Y. Yabe, "Fusion of Transformed Human Cells by Simian Retroviruses," *Gann*, vol. 71, June, 1980, pp. 367-371.

[132] P. Sonigo, C. Barker, E. Hunter, S. Wain-Hobson, "Nucleotide Sequence of Mason-Pfizer Monkey Virus: An Immuosuppressive D-Type Retrovirus," *Cell*, vol. 45, May 9, 1986, pp. 375-385.

[133] Indeed, cancer researchers tested the immunosuppressive properties of numerous viruses from both monkeys and humans in human cell cultures during this time period.

[134] An outbreak of the deadly West Nile virus in New York was blamed for 62 cases of encephalitis in 1999. Seven people died as a result of the outbreak, which caused a national panic. Parts of New York City were shut down so that officials could spray

pesticides in an effort to kill mosquitoes which were thought to be spreading the virus to humans. Mike Cooper, "West Nile virus RNA found in New York mosquitoes," *Reuters*, 3/9/00; Eric Lipton, "Virus Shuts Central Park; Wider Spraying Scheduled," *New York Times*, 7/25/00.

[135] C. M. Southam, L. Pillemer, "Serum Properdin Levels and Cancer Cell Homografts in Man," *Proceedings Soc. of Experimental Biology and Medicine (P.S.E.B.M.)*, vol. 96, p. 600.

[136] The authors noted: "The basis for this study was the finding of Southam et. al. that 'terminal cancer patients' can temporarily support the growth of subcutaneously implanted malignant human cells."

[137] Although a *New York Times* reporter [Altman] recently noted "it would be unethical to inject humans with a virus to prove that it can cause cancer," as documented in this work, scientists have conducted numerous experiments using just such a procedure. Lawrence K. Altman, "A Virus Associated With AIDS Is Linked To Appearance of a Common Blood Cancer," *New York Times*, 6/20/97.

[138] As Southam summarized his experiment, "It seemed reasonable to test this possibility by studying quantitatively the transplantability of syngeneic tumours under conditions which suppress or enhance immunological responses." J. Reiner, C. M. Southam, "Effect of Immunosuppression on First-Generation Isotransplantation of Chemically Induced Tumours in Mice," *Nature*, vol. 210, April 23, 1966, pp. 429-30.

[139] Some of the human patients used in the monkey virus experiment were undergoing immunosuppressive treatments with Cytoxan for their cancer: "Seventy-five percent of the patients had been given cytotoxic drugs, including cyclophosphamide (Cytoxan), 5-fluorodeoxyuridine, and 5-fluorouracil in full therapeutic doses." Researchers were able to study the injected cancer cell growth as a function of how long the immunosuppressive treatments had been previously halted: "[Cancer] Cells were inoculated into patients 1 to 31 days after drug administration was terminated, except for 2 patients who received their last dose of Cytoxan on the day implantation." F.

Jensen, H. Koprowski, J. S. Pagano, J. Ponten, R. G. Ravdin, "Autologous and Homologous Implantation of Human Cells Transformed In Vitro by Simian Virus 40," *Journal of the National Cancer Institute,* vol. 32, no. 4, April 1964, pp. 922-937.

[140] As Southam explained: "Such an investigation has been undertaken in this laboratory and the results obtained with cyclophosphamide ('Cytoxan') are sufficiently interesting and reliable to merit this preliminary report. Cyclophosphamide ('Cytoxan') was chosen for this study because its immunosuppressive effect had previously been demonstrated in a variety of experimental systems and because its pharmacological characteristics seem well suited to the objective." This chemical had the advantage: "This drug... acts very rapidly after systemic administration to initiate cytotoxic changes, including destruction of those cells responsible for immunological reactions." Conveniently, "if administration of the drug is stopped 24 h or more before a transplant is injected, it results in a host in which immunosuppression will continue for a considerable time, but in which there is no persistence of a cytotoxic drug which might inhibit the tumor transplant."

[141] The caption of Table 5 read: "Growth of nodules after homologous implantations of SV40-transformed cultures related to cell dosage and length of time spent in tissue culture after exposure to SV40." The subheading read: "Ratios represent number of sites showing growth of nodules over number of sites inoculated." F. Jensen, H. Koprowski, J. S. Pagano, J. Ponten, R. G. Ravdin, "Autologous and Homologous Implantation of Human Cells Transformed In Vitro by Simian Virus 40," *Journal of the National Cancer Institute,* vol. 32, no. 4, April 1964, pp. 922-937.

[142] See: G. A. Cole, K. V. Shah, "Experimental Simian Virus 40 Infection of Normal and Immunosuppressed Spider Monkeys," *Acta virol,* vol. 18, 1974, pp. 65-69.

[143] In this manner, researchers attempted to experimentally verify that the SV40 monkey virus fulfilled Koch's postulates in human cancer growth. This meant that for an agent to be responsible for a disease 1) it had to be present in all cases of the disease 2) it had to cause the disease when intentionally placed in healthy subjects

and 3) it had to be present in the intentionally infected subject. See: J. Cohen, "Fulfilling Koch's Postulates," *Nature*, vol. 266, 1994, p. 1647.

[144] J. T. Grace, Jr., E. A. Mirand, "Human Susceptibility to a Simian Tumor Virus," *Ann. N. Y. Acad. Sci.*, vol. 108, 1963, pp. 1123-1128.

[145] R. S. Metzgar, J. T. Grace, Jr., E. E. Sproul, "Immunological Studies of Subcutaneous Virus-Induced Histiocytomas In Primates," *Ann. N. Y. Acad. Sci.*, vol. 101, pp. 192-202.

[146] H. C. Chopra, M. M. Mason, "A New Virus in a Spontaneous Mammary Tumor of a Rhesus Monkey," *Cancer Research*, vol. 30, August 1970, pp. 2081-2086.

[147] J. Denner, V. Wunderlich, D. Bierwolf, "Suppression of Human Lymphocyte Mitogen Response By Proteins of the Type-D Retrovirus PMFV," *Int. J. Cancer*, vol. 37, 1986, pp. 311-316.

[148] H. Ogura, M. Ocho, T. Tanaka, T. Oda, "Susceptibility of Human Cultured Cells to Mason-Pfizer Monkey Virus," *Gann*, vol. 69, June, 1978, pp. 413-415.

[149] H. Ogura, T. Tanaka, M. Ocho, To Kuwata, T. Oda, "Detection of Mason-Pfizer Monkey Virus Infection by Syncytia Formation of Human Cells Doubly Transformed by Rous Sarcoma Virus and Simian Virus 40," *Archives of Virology*, vol. 57, 1978, pp. 195-198.

[150] H. Ogura, "Interactions Among Retroviruses Mason-Pfizer Monkey, Baboon Endogenous, Simian Sarcoma Virus-Associated and Murine Leukemia Detected by Virus-Mediated Cell Fusion Inhibition Assay," *Microbiol. Immunol.*, vol. 24, no. 8, 1980, pp. 761-763.

[151] See: J. Denner, V. Wunderlich, D. Bierwolf, "Suppression of Human Lymphocyte Mitogen Response By Proteins of the Type-D Retrovirus PMFV," *Int. J. Cancer*, vol. 37, 1986, pp. 311-316.

[152] A. M. Levine, "AIDS-Related Malignancies: the Emerging Epidemic," *Journal of the National Cancer Institute*, vol. 85, no. 17, September 1, 1993, p. 1392.

[153] Researchers have been systematically searching for such human cancer viruses for over 40 years. Up until the advent of the AIDS epidemic, this search had been in vain. The *New York*

Times summarized the overall situation in 1975 as follows: "... more than 100 different viruses have been proved capable of causing some kind of cancers in some animal species under some circumstances. Many viruses have been suggested as possible causative factors of some cancers in man, but no such case has been proved to date." Harold M. Schmeck, Jr. "Scientists Find Virus Linked to Human Leukemia; Diagnostic Value Seen," *New York Times*, 1/9/75.

[154] The source of Kaposi's sarcoma, the leading form of cancer that develops in immunosuppressed AIDS patients, has recently been traced to a type of herpes virus. Lawrence K. Altman, "Virus Linked To a Cancer Is Identified: Malignancy Is Found In Gay AIDS Patients," *New York Times*, 3/1/96.

[155] Cancer researchers had long theorized that human cancers could be caused by herpes viruses. In the 1970s, researchers wrote numerous papers speculating on the manner in which such viruses might cause human cancer. AIDS is providing the perfect research vehicle for proving these theories.

[156] Lawrence K. Altman, "A Virus Associated With AIDS Is Linked To Appearance of a Common Blood Cancer," *New York Times*, 6/20/97.

[157] D. T. Purtilo, "Opportunistic Cancers in Patients With Immunodeficiency Syndromes," *Arch. Pathol. Lab. Med.*, vol. 111, Dec. 1987, p. 1123.

[158] V. Beral, H. Jaffe and R. Weiss, "Cancer Surveys: Cancer, HIV and AIDS," *Eur. J. Cancer*, vol. 27, no. 8, 1991, p. 1057.

[159] J. Iscovich, P. Boffetta, R. Winkelmann, P. Brennan, E. Azizi, "Classic Kaposi's Sarcoma in Jews Living in Israel, 1961-1989: A Population-Based Incidence Study, *AIDS*, 1998, vol. 12, p. 2068.

[160] Lawrence K. Altman, "Rare Cancer Seen in 41 Homosexuals," *New York Times*, July 3, 1981.

[161] Lawrence K. Altman, "Surviving With AIDS Is One Problem, Cancer Is Yet Another," *New York Times*, 5/6/97.

[162] D. T. Purtilo, "Opportunistic Cancers in Patients With Immunodeficiency Syndromes," *Arch. Pathol. Lab. Med.*, vol. 111, Dec. 1987, p. 1129.

[163] V. Beral, H. Jaffe and R. Weiss, "Cancer Surveys: Cancer, HIV and AIDS," *Eur. J. Cancer*, vol. 27, no. 8, 1991, pp. 1058.

[164] R. A. Good, "Relations Between Immunity and Malignancy," *Proc. Nat. Acad. Sci USA*, vol. 69, no. 4, April 1972, pp. 1026-1032.

[165] H. Temin, "The RNA Tumor Viruses—Background and Foreground, *Proc. Nat. Acad. Sci USA*, vol. 69, no. 4, April 1972, pp. 1016-1020.

[166] G. Klein, "Herpes viruses and Oncogenesis," *Proc. Nat. Acad. Sci USA*, vol. 69 no. 4, April 1972, pp. 1056-1064.

[167] S. Matsui, J. Ahlers, A. Vortmeyer, M. Terabe, T. Tsukui, D. Carbone, L. Liotta, J. Berzofsky, "A Model for CD8+ CTL Tumor Immunosurveillance and Regulation of Tumor Escape by CD4 T Cells Through an Effect on Quality of CTL," *Journal of Immunology*, vol. 163, no.1, July 1, 1999, pp. 184-193.

[168] Y. N. Vaishnav, F. Wong-Staal, "The Biochemistry of AIDS," *Annu. Rev. Biochem.* 1991, vol. 60, p. 580.

[169] Andrew Pollack, "Scientists Enlist H.I.V. To Fight Other Ills," *New York Times*, 1/19/99.

[170] In 1990, the prestigious journal *Science* published an incredible technical paper by a group of researchers (including the infamous Robert Gallo—co-discoverer of the HIV) describing in detail their successful attempts at *creating* a "super" AIDS virus with greatly enhanced infectious properties. This new and highly dangerous AIDS virus was deliberately engineered—through the sophisticated use of immunosuppression and a mixing of human and animal viruses—to infect a greater number of cell types than the "natural" AIDS virus had been capable of infecting. Additionally, this newly engineered AIDS virus was thought to be transmissible through the air, as the new virus was made capable of infecting cells of the respiratory tract. See: P. Lusso, F. Veronese, B. Ensoli, G. Franchini, C. Jemma, S. E. DeRocco, V. S. Kalyanaraman, R. C. Gallo, "Expanded HIV-1 Cellular Tropism by Phenotypic Mixing with Murine Endogenous Retroviruses," *Science*, vol. 247, 16 February 1990, pp. 848-852.

[171] As Jean Marx summarized in *Science*, "As a result, the AIDS virus, also known as HIV-1 (for human immunodeficiency virus

1), acquires some new biological characteristics, including the ability to reproduce much more rapidly than it normally does and to infect new kinds of cells." J. Marx, "Concerns Raised About Mouse Models for AIDS," *Science*, vol. 247 1990, p. 809.

[172] Lawrence K. Altman, "The Doctor's World: AIDS Research Yields Clues Linking Viruses and Cancer," *New York Times*, 4/14/98.

[173] This is one of the reasons cancer researchers were so intensely interested in determining whether animal cancer viruses could cause human cancer. If animal cancer viruses were responsible for some human cancers, and vaccines existed for these viruses, then animal cancer vaccines might be directly used as human cancer vaccines.

[174] In a similar manner, the cowpox virus found in cattle was used as an early vaccine against human smallpox.

[175] C. M. Southam, "Studies of Host Defense Against Human Cancer," *Indian J Cancer*, vol. 4, no. 1, March 1967, p. 13.

[176] W. L. Drew, L. Mintz, R. C. Miner, M. Sands, B. Ketterer, "Prevalence of Cytomegalovirus Infection in Homosexual Men," *Journal of Infectious Diseases*, vol. 143, no. 2, Feb. 1981, pp. 188-192.

[177] Additionally, researchers monitoring homosexuals with HIV and the herpesvirus which is thought to cause Kaposi's sarcoma are able to verify that the herpesvirus is a key factor in the cancer by comparing cancer rates in HIV positive blood transfusion recipients without the herpesvirus. D. Whitby, M. Howard, M. Tenant-Flowers, N. Brink, A. Copas, C. Boshoff, T. Hatzioannou, F. Suggett, D. Aldam, A. Denton, R. Miller, I. Weller, R. Weiss, R. Tedder. T. Schulz, "Detection of Kaposi Sarcoma Associated Herpesvirus in Peripheral blood of HIV-Infected Individuals and Progression to Kaposi's Sarcoma," *The Lancet*, vol. 346, Sept. 23, 1995, pp. 799-802.

[178] Such an experiment as that just proposed to explain why gays may have been targeted for experimentation might be considered a more sophisticated version of previously published experiments in which formerly cancer-free human patients, which had undergone organ transplants from cancerous donors, became

infected with cancer. Researchers were able to manipulate and monitor the cancer growth in these patients by withholding or administering immunosuppressive treatments. (Gross) In a unique twist on this phenomenon, cancer researchers may be able to modulate cancer growth by starting anti-immunosuppressive treatments in AIDS patients. This is due to the fact that anti-HIV medication may only partially restore the immune system health of AIDS victims. Thus, by monitoring cancer rates in AIDS patients before and after AIDS-related drug therapies, researchers may gain further insight into exactly which T-cell subsets actually assist in preventing cancer. See L. Gross, "Transmission of Cancer in Man," *Cancer*, vol. 28, pp. 785-788; Lawrence Altman, "THE DOCTOR'S WORLD: AIDS Research Yields Clues Linking Viruses and Cancer, *New York Times*, 4/14/98.

[179] Establishment researchers postulating that HIV derives from SIV (through a monkey bite or the consumption of contaminated monkey meat) consistently neglect to inform the public that numerous experiments have been conducted by the cancer research establishment over the years in which simian cancer and tumor viruses were systematically injected directly into human test subjects in successful attempts to induce tumors. If the simian immunodeficiency virus (SIV) was an unknown virus at the time these experiments were conducted, there is no way researchers could have screened these viruses out of their experimental monkey virus injections in human subjects. This systematic injection of human test subjects with monkey viruses would appear to be a much more likely candidate for the origin of the AIDS epidemic than the "monkey bite," or related theories. Also of concern is the fact that in the 1950s and 60s millions of people were given polio vaccines contaminated with simian cancer viruses. These vaccines could also have been a source for SIVs. For a discussion of this theory, see: Tom Curtis, "The Origin of AIDS," *Rolling Stone*, March 19th, 1992 pp. 54-108; and B. F. Elswood, R. B. Stricker, "Polio Vaccines and the Origin of AIDS," *Medical Hypothesis*, vol. 42, 1994, pp. 347-354.

[180] Such covert international experimentation is hardly unprecedented. The U.S. government completed similar covert

and unethical experiments on an international scale during the height of the MKULTRA drug testing programs (which were exposed in congressional investigations in the 1970s).

[181] "The United States has become increasingly dependent on mineral imports from developing countries in recent decades, and this trend is likely to continue. The location of known reserves of higher-grade ores of most minerals favors increasing dependence of all industrialized regions on imports from less developed countries." *National Security Study Memorandum 200*, "Implications Of Worldwide Population Growth For U.S. Security And Overseas Interests," December 10, 1974 [Declassified 7/3/89], p. 37.

[182] *National Security Study Memorandum 200*, "Implications Of Worldwide Population Growth For U.S. Security And Overseas Interests," December 10, 1974 [Declassified 7/3/89], p. 43.

[183] "Implications of Worldwide Population Growth for U.S. Security and Overseas Interests," *National Security Study Memorandum 200*, December, 10, 1974, Confidential (Declassified 7/3/89), p. 18.

[184] In the words of the NSC study, "*a current danger of the highest magnitude calling for urgent measures ...*"

[185] As a follow-up memo authorized: "The President, therefore, assigns to the Chairman, NSC Under Secretaries Committee, the responsibility to define and develop policy in the population field and to coordinate its implementation beyond the NSSM 200 response." Brent Scowcroft, "Implications Of Worldwide Population Growth For U.S. Security And Overseas Interests," *National Security Decision Memorandum 314*, copied to the Chairman of Joint Chiefs of Staff, and Director of CIA, November 26, 1975 [Confidential, Declassified].

[186] Due to exorbitant costs and poor health infrastructures typically found in the Third World, progress recently made in fighting the diseases caused by AIDS with protease inhibitors (through the so-called AIDS cocktail) in the developed world is problematic on a global basis. A far cheaper method of treatment will have to be found to prevent millions of AIDS-related deaths in the developing world. As Youssef M. Ibrahim, writing in the

New York Times, summarized, "barring a miracle in the pharmaceutical industry that discovers radical remedies for AIDS, countries like Botswana and Zimbabwe will loose [sic] as much as a fifth of their population within the next decade." Youssef M. Ibrahim, "AIDS Is Slashing Africa's Population, U.N. Survey Finds," *New York Times*, 10/28/98.

[187] The depopulation effects of AIDS are projected to be especially severe in sub-Saharan Africa where some nations are projected to lose one quarter of their populations due to the virus. This development may fulfill the population planners' goals for Third World depopulation without the use of more traditional means of population control.

[188] CNN, "Life expectancy in Africa cut short by AIDS," March 18, 1999; CNN Web posted at: 12:24 p.m. EST (1724 GMT).

[189] This was relayed by George Bush in 1969 during the Republican Task Force on Resources and Population hearings, which he headed.

[190] As summarized in the declassified study: "Under the U.N. medium projection variant, by the year 2000 the population of less developed countries would double, rising from 2.5 billion to 5.0 billion. Thus, by the year 2000 ... over 90 percent of the annual increment to world population would occur there." *National Security Study Memorandum 200*, "Implications Of Worldwide Population Growth For U.S. Security And Overseas Interests," December 10, 1974 [Declassified 7/3/89], p. 17.

[191] Editorial, "The Global Plague of AIDS," *New York Times*, 4/23/00.

[192] AP, "Report Expects AIDS to Depress Africa's Fast Population Growth," *New York Times*, 7/3/96.

[193] AP, "Report Expects AIDS to Depress Africa's Fast Population Growth," *New York Times*, 7/3/96.

[194] AP, "Facts About AIDS in Africa," Filed at 11:26 a.m. EST, By The Associated Press January 10, 2000.

[195] 91% of the AIDS related deaths in the world have been in only 34 sub-Saharan countries. The *New York Times* notes that, "In Botswana, the hardest hit country in sub-Saharan Africa, life expectancy, which stood at 61 years only five years ago, has

dropped to 47 and is expected to drop to 41 between 2000 and 2005. In Zimbabwe, where one of every five adults is infected, the high mortality rate is significantly reducing the country's population and its growth, from 3.3 percent a year between 1980 and 1985 to 1.4 percent now and a projection of less than 1 percent beginning in 2000." Youssef M. Ibrahim, "AIDS Is Slashing Africa's Population, U.N. Survey Finds," *New York Times*, 10/28/98.

[196] Jane Perlez, "AIDS in Africa Is Seen Halting Population Rise," *New York Times*, 6/22/92.

[197] Ibid.

[198] The development of viruses for biowarfare whose infectious properties sound remarkably like those of HIV were foreshadowed in the late 1960s in various government publications. For example, in the *Congressional Record* on June 25, 1970 (p. 21395) excerpts were printed from a report of the Subcommittee on National Security Policy and Scientific Developments of the House Foreign Relations Committee which contained the following warning:

> Secondly, on the immediate horizon are modern developments in molecular genetics which could result in manmade viruses for which there would be no natural immunities and against which no reasonable defense could be mounted.

During the early debate over initiating a genetic bioweapons research program through the civilian sector, a Dr. MacArthur appeared before a Congressional investigative committee (Department of Defense Appropriations for 1970) and presented a prepared statement which revealed some interesting information about the line of research that was being considered. MacArthur's statement contained the following startling prediction:

> Within the next 5 to 10 years, it would probably be possible to make a new infective microorganism which could differ in certain

important aspects from any known disease-causing organisms. Most important of these is that it might be refractory to the immunological and therapeutic processes upon which we depend to maintain our relative freedom from infectious disease. [emphasis added]

Roughly ten years from the time this "prediction" was made, the AIDS virus began destroying the immunological processes of millions of human beings, thereby making it impossible for them to maintain their "relative freedom from infectious disease."

[199] The viral cancer research community and the biowarfare community have been working hand-in-glove for several decades. In fact, the biowarfare labs at Fort Detrick were converted into a National Cancer Institute cancer research facility–which, it was announced–would work with viruses thought to be capable of causing human cancer. As Harold Schmeck noted in the *New York Times* in 1972: "The cancer institute's operation at Fort Detrick will be located primarily in the 'high security area' of the former biological warfare research facility." The *Times* also noted that, "work at Ft. Detrick would include research on known cancer viruses of animals as well as some of the viruses suspected of roles in human cancer." See: Harold M. Schmeck, Jr. "Litton to Run Cancer Research Lab," *New York Times*, 6/25/72.

[200] Barton Gellman, "The World Shunned Signs of Coming Plague," *Washington Post*, 7/7/00.

[201] The Associated Press, "Gore Announces Money To Fight AIDS," *New York Times*, 1/10/00.

[202] See, for example, the recent final reports of the Clinton administration's President's Advisory Committee on Human Radiation Experiments (900 pages long) or the Final Report of the Committee on Veterans' Affairs United States Senate; Hearing, "Is Military Research Hazardous to Veterans' Health? Lessons from the Cold War, the Persian Gulf, and Today."

[203] These exercises may have killed tens of thousands of Chinese civilians. Nicholas D. Kristof, writing in the *New York Times*, summarized these experiments as follows:

"The Japanese Army regularly conducted field tests to see whether biological warfare would work outside the laboratory. Planes dropped plague-infected fleas over Ningbo in eastern China and over Changde in north-central China, and plague outbreaks were later reported ... Japanese troops also dropped cholera and typhoid cultures in wells and ponds, but the results were often counterproductive. In 1942 germ warfare specialists distributed dysentery, cholera and typhoid in Zhejiang Province in China, but Japanese soldiers became ill and 1,700 died of the diseases, scholars say."

Nicholas D Kristof, "Japan Confronting Gruesome War Atrocity," *New York Times*, 3/17/95.

[204] As the *New York Times* recently put it, with respect to the histories of these war criminals: "Japanese and American documents show that the United States helped cover up the human experimentation. Instead of putting the ringleaders on trial it gave them stipends." Ed Regis summarized this disgraceful development as follows: "There could be no doubt, at this point, that the principal Japanese germ warfare figures were war criminals of the greatest magnitude, on the order of Josef Mengele and other Nazi doctors who had performed experiments of unimaginable cruelty on concentration camp prisoners during World War II. The Soviets, indeed, wanted to prosecute the Japanese Unit 731 hierarchy for their role in such crimes, yet the American biological scientists, in their rush to get the scientific data, showed no evidence of being held back by any moral, legal, or other constraints, and willingly promised immunity to Shiro Ishii and all the rest in order to get it." Nicholas D. Kristof, "Japan Confronting Gruesome War Atrocity," *New York Times*, 3/17/95; Ed Regis, *The Biology of Doom: The History of America's Secret Germ Warfare Project*, (New York: Henry Holt and Company, 1999), p. 129. See also: Peter Williams, David Wallace, *Unit 731,*

Japan's Secret Biological Warfare in World War II (New York: The Free Press, 1989); Sheldon Harris, *Factories of Death: Japanese Biological Warfare, 1932-45, and the American Cover-Up*, (London: Routledge, 1994)

[205] Some of these Nazi doctors were acting as consultants to American military agencies while these agencies experimented on thousands of U.S. soldiers at Edgewood Arsenal in Maryland. These experiments duplicated those conducted in Nazi concentration camps and even used gas chambers to expose American soldiers to deadly nerve gases that the Nazis developed during the war. (Ten tons of these gases were shipped to America after the war.) Linda Hunt, *Secret Agenda: The United States Government, Nazi Scientists, and Project Paperclip, 1945-1990*, (New York: St. Martin's Press, 1991), p. 132.

[206] Kurt Waldheim, a member of several Nazi organizations and a Nazi intelligence officer, eventually became the Secretary General of the U.N., and later, the president of Austria (with the help of the U.S. State Department and the U.S. Representative to the U.N.–George Bush). Robert Herzstein, *Waldheim, The Missing Years*, (New York: Paragon House, 1989), p. 267.

[207] Associated Press, "German Doctor, an Ex-Nazi, Gives Up International Post," *New York Times*, 1/24/93.

[208] Dr. Futaki (head of the tuberculosis research effort at Unit 731) became the president of S. J. Company Ltd.; Dr. Hayakawa became a manager of the Hayakawa Medical Company; Dr. Kanazawa (who did tick research for biowarfare applications) headed up a research section at Takeda Pharmaceutical Company. Dr. Tanaka (who mass-produced fleas for biological warfare delivery) became director of Osaka Municipal University's School of Medicine (and was later given an Order of the Rising Sun), Dr. Yamanaka became the dean of the Osaka Medical School; Dr. Yoshimura (who directed frostbite experiments where people were deliberately frozen to death) became president of the Kyoto Prefectural Medical College and president of the Japanese Meteorological Society; Dr. Okamoto (a pathology squad leader who conducted vivisection experiments) became medical director of Kinki University at Osaka and director of the University of

Kyoto's medical department; Dr. Ishikawa (a pathologist at Unit 731) became president of the medical school at Kanazawa University. Peter Williams, David Wallace, *Unit 731, Japan's Secret Biological Warfare in World War II* (New York: The Free Press, 1989), pp. 236-241.

[209] See: Peter Williams, David Wallace, *Unit 731, Japan's Secret Biological Warfare in World War II*, (New York: The Free Press, 1989), pp. 236-241; Sheldon Harris, *Factories of Death: Japanese Biological Warfare, 1932-45, and the American Cover-Up*, (London: Routledge, 1994), p. 133.

[210] These experiments used immune system modulating methods in combination with the deliberate infection of healthy prisoners with deadly bacteria and viruses including yellow fever, smallpox, typhus, paratyphus, cholera and diphtheria. These tests were designed to test the vaccines developed by German pharmaceuticals corporations. For a description of these vaccine experiments, see: TRIALS OF WAR CRIMINALS BEFORE THE NUERNBERG MILITARY TRIBUNALS, Volume II, (Washington D.C.: U.S. Government Printing Office, October 1946-April 1949), p. 178.

[211] If these particular criminal elements *were* involved in infecting large portions of the globe with immunosuppressive viruses as part of an AIDS experiment, such experimentation could be seen as merely the continuation of their criminal wartime research in peacetime with a much larger experimental base.

[212] Such field trials may have included the use of biological warfare by the U.S. during the Korean War. For a discussion of this possibility, see Sheldon Harris, *Factories of Death*, (London: Routledge, 1994) pp. 230-232.

[213] G. W. Christopher, T. J. Cieslak, J. A. Pavlin, E. M. Eitzen, "Biological Warfare: A Historical Perspective," *JAMA*, August 6, 1997, Vol. 278, No. 5, pp. 413.

[214] Using researchers from the biowarfare establishment for allegedly humanitarian purposes had been recommended in 1970 by a House Foreign Relations Committee: "Every possible effort should be made to retain former BW facilities and personnel, turning them to the solution of environmental problems for the

benefit of all Americans and, indeed, all mankind." "Report of the Subcommittee on National Security Policy and Scientific Developments of the House Foreign Relations Committee," *Congressional Record*, June 25, 1970, p. 21396.

[215] Quoted in "Biological Testing Involving Human Subjects by the Department of Defense, 1977," *Hearings Before the Subcommittee on Health and Scientific Research of the Committee on Human Resources United States Senate*, 1977, p. 266.

[216] "Chemical-Biological Warfare, US Policies and International Effects," *Report of the Subcommittee on National Security Policy and Scientific Developments of the Committee on Foreign Affairs, House of Representatives*, May 16, 1970, p. 127.

[217] Dalrymple, "DoD-Sponsored Virus Vaccine Development: An Investigator's Perspective," *Annals of the New York Academy of Sciences*, vol. 666, p. 210.

[218] Some personnel from labs that were involved in the San Francisco open air tests using simulants (e.g. Naval Biosciences Laboratory) were also used in this cancer research program.

[219] R. Hatch, "Cancer Warfare," *Covert Action Information Bulletin*, Number 39 (Winter 1991-92), pp. 14, 15.

[220] Harold M. Schmeck, Jr. "Litton to Run Cancer Research Lab," *New York Times*, 6/25/72.

[221]The *Guardian Unlimited* reported the following in October 2001: "The Pentagon has approved the development of a genetically modified 'super-anthrax' bacteria to test US defences against biological attack, overriding concerns that the research could violate a 1972 germ warfare treaty, it was reported yesterday." Julian Borger, "Pentagon approves super strain: US developing more potent anthrax to test vaccine," 10/24/01.

[222] "Project MKULTRA, The CIA's Program of Research In Behavioral Modification," *Joint Hearing Before the Select Committee on Intelligence and the Subcommittee on Health and Scientific Research of the Committee on Human Resources*, Ninety-Fifth Congress, First Session, August 3, 1977, p. 389.

[223] "Project MKULTRA, The CIA's Program of Research In Behavioral Modification," p. 391.

[224] As revealed by the *New York Times*: "In the early years of the cold war, a systematic effort to gain knowledge of the effects of radiation from experiments on human subjects was secretly planned at the highest levels of the United States Government." P. Hilts, "Panel Finds Wide Debate in 40's On the Ethics of Radiation Tests," *New York Times*, 10/12/94

[225] Associated Press, "U.S. Continues Defensive Germ Warfare Research," *New York Times,* 9/7/82.

[226] J. M. Dalrymple, "DoD-Sponsored Virus Vaccine Development: An Investigator's Perspective," in *The Microbiologist and Biological Defense Research: Ethics, Politics, and International Security*, Annals of the New York Academy of Sciences, vol. 666, p. 203.

[227] Ibid., p. 218.

[228] Paul Lewis, "U.N. Agencies to Combine Efforts Against AIDS," *New York Times*, 1/23/94.

[229] "Convinced that the global spread of AIDS is reaching catastrophic dimensions, the Clinton administration has formally designated the disease for the first time as a threat to U.S. national security that could topple foreign governments, touch off ethnic wars and undo decades of work in building free-market democracies abroad." Barton Gellman, "AIDS Is Declared Threat to Security," *Washington Post*, 4/30/00.